Concussion

What Do I Do Now?

SERIES CO-EDITORS-IN-CHIEF

Lawrence C. Newman, MD
Director of the Headache Division
Professor of Neurology
New York University Langone
New York, New York

Morris Levin, MD
Director of the Headache Center
Professor of Neurology
University of California, San Francisco
San Francisco, California

OTHER VOLUMES IN THE SERIES

Concussion

Brian Hainline, MD
NCAA Chief Medical Officer, Indianapolis, IN
Clinical Professor of Neurology
Indiana University School of Medicine, Indianapolis, IN
New York University School of Medicine, New York, NY

Lindsey J. Gurin, MD
Clinical Assistant Professor of Neurology, Psychiatry,
and Rehabilitation Medicine
New York University School of Medicine, New York, NY

Daniel M. Torres, MD
Clinical Assistant Professor of Neurology
New York University School of Medicine, New York, NY

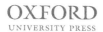

OXFORD
UNIVERSITY PRESS

OXFORD
UNIVERSITY PRESS

Oxford University Press is a department of the University of Oxford. It furthers
the University's objective of excellence in research, scholarship, and education
by publishing worldwide. Oxford is a registered trade mark of Oxford University
Press in the UK and certain other countries.

Published in the United States of America by Oxford University Press
198 Madison Avenue, New York, NY 10016, United States of America.

CIP data is on file at the Library of Congress
ISBN 978–0–19–093744–7

9 8 7 6 5 4 3 2 1

Printed by Marquis, Canada

Contents

Foreword

I am deeply honored that my neurology colleagues at NYU Langone have asked me to write the foreword for their new book on concussion as part of the series "What Do I Do Now?" Dr. Brian Hainline, the first chief medical officer at the NCAA, has teamed with two NYU concussion experts, Drs. Lindsey Gurin and Daniel Torres, to create a practical and timely book on how to manage the various problems that arise following concussion. Dr. Hainline, a recognized thought leader in the field, brings a unique background to this endeavor as a former NCAA Division 1 athlete in tennis, as well as a neurologist who has specialized in sports neurology for over three decades. Dr. Hainline has also been on the front line of this area as we gather longitudinal information about the natural history of concussion and its consequences. Dr. Gurin has trained in both neurology and psychiatry, and has a special interest in the cognitive issues that arise after head injury. Dr. Torres is a clinical neurologist who has dedicated his expertise to this area. The book will be welcomed by practitioners in many areas of medicine, as head trauma touches many fields, including neurology, ophthalmology, neurosurgery, sports medicine, orthopedics, and rehabilitation medicine—to just name a few.

In 2012, when I arrived to serve as chair of neurology at NYU Langone, the area of concussion was just beginning to be widely recognized as a major cause of morbidity. The problem of repetitive head injury was acknowledged long ago, but the actual consequences had been poorly appreciated by physicians, other practitioners in the field, and the public. A new multidisciplinary service was created at NYU Langone Health to enhance the clinical, educational, and research efforts in this rapidly evolving field. The demand to see patients was extreme, and the need to disseminate information about how to manage them even greater. We initiated frequent case conferences and journal clubs to discuss the challenging problems arising from concussion and other forms of mild traumatic brain injury. This book is, in part, the product of those discussions as well as the vast clinical experience of the authors.

In the preface, the authors outline the purpose of this book as a simple guide that "cuts to the chase" regarding diagnosis and management of concussion. Using individual case examples, the authors walk through the presentations of concussion, including what to do on the field of play and how to deal with more complicated situations, including cervical spine injury, or how to manage the patient who has evolving neurological signs. Each chapter ends with the key take-home points, and the authors provide a boatload of tables and other helpful forms. The reader is provided with discussions on how to evaluate the patient who worsens at one hour—or how to approach the patient with continued symptoms. Importantly, the authors provide guidance on how to manage the expectations for recovery. Persistent symptoms are, unfortunately, common for a subset of patients; the reader is guided through specific problems that follow concussion, such as headache, sleep impairment, depression, anxiety, emotional dysregulation, autonomic conditions, vestibular dysfunction, visual impairment, and pituitary dysregulation. The third section of the book is dedicated to other medical and societal considerations associated with the topic of concussion. The authors tackle the issues of hiding concussion, challenging interactions with coaches, retirement from contact sports, and the legal concerns that may follow concussion. In the final sections, contemporary discussions about the long-term consequences of repetitive head injury, such as chronic traumatic encephalopathy, are examined. The book is a quick and enjoyable read, either on an individual issue or as a complete overview of the timely topic of concussion.

The book will appeal to a wide audience, including the many stakeholders of the concussion story, such as athletes, parents, physicians in virtually all areas of medicine, therapists, athletic trainers, coaches, and the lay public. The field of concussion is evolving rapidly; the issues not only are medically complex, but also have great impact on our society and how we view sport in general. Drs. Hainline, Gurin, and Torres have brought all of these issues to the forefront. Their wisdom on manifestations and management will be greatly appreciated by the many who want to know what to do now!

Steven Galetta, MD
Philip Moskowitz Professor and Chair of Neurology
Professor of Ophthalmology
New York University School of Medicine
New York, NY

Preface

It is estimated that sport-related concussions account for 1.6–3.8 million traumatic brain injuries that occur annually in the United States. Concussion has become an increasingly recognized public health concern, and there has been a recent dramatic shift in the diagnosis and management of sport-related concussion. Previously, concussion was not always considered a medical concern, with little uniformity in medical management guidelines. Indeed, it was not until 2014 that concussion education became a mandatory requirement in neurology residency training, and such training is not synchronized with concussion training in other medical specialties.

This book is an attempt to present a concise, simple, and clear format for understanding and managing concussion, and is divided into four sections. Part I provides a broad overview of the manifestations and management of acute concussion. Most individuals who sustain a concussion recover, and emerging information tells us that concussion is a treatable condition. The earlier concussion is treated, the better the outcome. Part II focuses on manifestations and management of persistent symptoms among those who do not recover following a concussion. Those with persistent symptoms are too often erroneously diagnosed as having "post-concussion syndrome"—a term that is no longer medically acceptable. Emerging information tells us that concussion often manifests in different clinical profiles, and these profiles can be managed both acutely and in the longer term. Part III focuses on medical/societal considerations of concussion, exploring topics such as the culture of concussion safety and emerging information regarding repetitive head impact exposure. Part IV reviews possible long-term sequelae of concussion, including possible long-term sequelae of repetitive head impact exposure. Considerable scientific and emotional debate continues about the long-term sequelae of concussion. There is even debate that repetitive head impact exposure, not concussion, may be a better indicator of long-term sequelae.

We hope that this book provides a clear picture of this rapidly evolving field of medicine. Because there is such a gap in education about concussion, even among specialists such as neurologists, we believe that this book is suitable for all physicians and clinicians who may treat individuals with concussion, plus sports stakeholders, parents, and the media. Although we make our best attempt to wrestle with emerging information and present concrete management guidance, this book should not be interpreted as a clinical practice guideline or legal standard of care. Individual management always depends on the facts and circumstances specific to each individual case.

PART I

Manifestations and Management of Acute Concussion

1   Acute Concussion in the Emergency Department (Mary fell off her bike)

A 15-year-old girl presented to the Emergency Department following a head injury. She had been riding her bicycle and was wearing a helmet, but she was practicing riding her bike with no hands. She lost control, and when she fell from her bike, the side of her head struck the concrete pavement. Two of her friends observed the accident; both noted that she was motionless for less than one minute, and when she tried to stand up she appeared uncoordinated. She complained immediately of a headache, and she was taken to the Emergency Department by ambulance. Once in the Emergency Department, she had no symptoms other than a headache.

What do you do now?

ACUTE CONCUSSION IN THE EMERGENCY DEPARTMENT

There are over 3.8 million traumatic brain injuries in the United States each year, accounting for approximately 2.5 million Emergency Department visits. Most of these injuries are mild traumatic brain injuries. The terms "concussion" and "mild traumatic brain injury" are used interchangeably, but they are not the same thing. Mild traumatic brain injury is nonspecifically defined as a head injury that results in a Glasgow Coma Scale score between 13 and 15, assessed 30 minutes post-injury (Table 1.1).

For concussion, however, there are over 45 working definitions, and none provides objective biomarkers. In other words, concussion diagnosis is based on symptoms with no defining pathophysiologic profile for definitive diagnosis. The Concussion in Sport Group has provided an updated definition of concussion every 4 years for the past 20 years (Box 1.1). In the Emergency Department, the most commonly accepted definition of concussion stems from the Centers for Disease Control and Prevention, with

TABLE 1.1 **Glasgow Coma Scale**

Response	Scale	Score
Eye Opening Response	Eyes open spontaneously	4 points
	Eyes open to verbal command, speech, or shout	3 points
	Eyes open to pain (not applied to face)	2 points
	No eye opening	1 point
Verbal Response	Oriented	5 points
	Confused conversation, but able to answer questions	4 points
	Inappropriate responses, words discernible	3 points
	Incomprehensible sounds or speech	2 points
	No verbal response	1 point
Motor Response	Obeys commands for movement	6 points
	Purposeful movement to painful stimulus	5 points
	Withdraws from pain	4 points
	Abnormal flexion, decorticate posture	3 points
	Extensor response, decerebrate posture	2 points
	No motor response	1 point

Minor Brain Injury = 13–15 points; Moderate Brain Injury = 9–12 points; Severe Brain Injury = 3–8 points.

> BOX 1.1. **Concussion in Sport Group Definition of Concussion**
>
> Sport-related concussion (SRC) is a traumatic brain injury induced by biomechanical forces. Several common features that may be utilized in clinically defining the nature of a concussion head injury include the following:
>
> - SRC may be caused either by a direct blow to the head, face, or neck, or a blow elsewhere on the body with an impulsive force transmitted to the head.
> - SRC typically results in the rapid onset of short-lived impairment of neurological function that resolves spontaneously. However, in some cases, signs and symptoms evolve over a number of minutes to hours.
> - SRC may result in neuropathological changes, but the acute clinical signs and symptoms largely reflect a functional disturbance rather than a structural injury and, as such, no abnormality is seen on standard structural neuroimaging studies.
> - SRC results in a range of clinical signs and symptoms that may or may not involve loss of consciousness. Resolution of the clinical and cognitive features typically follows a sequential course. However, in some cases symptoms may be prolonged.
> - The clinical signs and symptoms cannot be explained by drug, alcohol, or medication use, other injuries (cervical injuries, peripheral vestibular dysfunction, etc.) or other comorbidities (e.g., psychological factors or coexisting medical conditions).

primary characteristics including the following: (1) an alteration in brain function caused by an external force—direct or indirect; (2) confusion or disorientation, loss of consciousness for less than 30 minutes, post-traumatic amnesia for less than 24 hours, or transient neurologic abnormalities; and (3) Glasgow Coma Scale score of between 13 and 15, assessed 30 minutes post-injury.

There is no uniform national protocol to evaluate concussion in the Emergency Department. In part, this is because the primary function of an

> ### BOX 1.2. **"Red Flags" for Ordering a Brain CT Scan**
>
> Focal neurologic findings
> Intoxication from alcohol or drugs
> Ongoing altered mental status, including irritability, confusion, change in personality/behavior
> Repeated vomiting
> Progressive worsening headache
> Seizures
> Trauma over temporal-parietal lesion (raises suspicion for epidural hematoma)
> Positive blood biomarker of C-terminal hydrolase-L1 (UCH-L1)

Emergency Department visit is to triage severe or life-threatening injuries versus minor injuries. Such triage includes deciding whether brain imaging studies should be obtained. The "red flags" for obtaining a brain imaging study are listed in Box 1.2. Importantly, a negative brain computed tomography (CT) scan is expected in concussion. It is also important to assess for associated injuries, especially to the cervical spine. Focal cervical pain should raise suspicion for a cervical spine evaluation.

Management of concussion in the Emergency Department should focus primarily on educating the patient and family about concussion, and assuring a proper and graduated return to activity. Most patients with a concussion can be discharged from the Emergency Department on the same day. The three most common mistakes in discharge instructions are as follows: (1) providing unsatisfactory education regarding expectations of concussion recovery; (2) providing unsatisfactory instructions regarding the importance of graduated exercise and return to activity; and (3) providing unsatisfactory instructions regarding the importance of supervised follow-up. A breakdown in any of the steps is associated with prolonged concussion recovery, persistent concussion symptoms, or both.

· Concussion evaluations are common in the Emergency Department.
· Brain CT scans are only required when "red flags" are present.
· A negative brain CT scan is expected in concussion.
· Discharge instructions should emphasize education about expectations of recovery, graduated return to activity, and supervised follow-up.

Further Reading

1) Wright DW, Bazarian JJ. Emergency department evaluation of the concussed athlete. In Hainline B, Stern RA (Eds.), *Sports Neurology*, San Diego: Elsevier BV, 2018, pp 81–90.

2) Ruff RM, Iverson GL, Barth JT, et al. Recommendations for diagnosing a mild traumatic brain injury: a National Academy of Neuropsychology education paper. *Arch Clin Neuropsychol* 2009;24:3–10.

3) McCrory P, Meeuwisse W, Dvorak J, et al. Consensus statement on concussion in sport—the 5th international conference on concussion in sport held in Berlin, October 2016. *Br J Sports Med* 2017;51:838–847.

4) Seabury SA, Guadette E, Goldman DP, et al. Assessment of follow-up care after emergency department presentation for mild traumatic brain injury and concussion: results from the TRACK-TBI study. *JAMA Network Open* 2018;1:1–13. doi:10.1001/jamanetworkopen.2018.0210.

5) Morrison L, Taylor R, Mercuri M, et al. Examining Canada's return visits to the emergency department after a concussion. *Canadian J Emerg Med* 2019;5:1–5. doi:10.1017/cem.2019.22. [Epub ahead of print]

2 Acute Concussion on the Field of Play
(Jane does not look right after trying to head the ball)

A 20-year-old female college soccer player was attempting to head a soccer ball when she collided headfirst with a player from the opposing team. She immediately felt dizzy and seemed to stumble, walking toward the opposing team's sideline. The athletic trainer on the sideline witnessed the event and immediately evaluated the athlete. The evaluation took place in a relatively quiet place, away from the sideline. The athlete was not allowed to return to play that day.

What do you do now?

ACUTE CONCUSSION ON THE FIELD OF PLAY

Concussion is a risk factor in all sports, especially contact and collision sports. The sideline assessment of possible sport-related concussion has evolved considerably over time. Although several return-to-play guidelines were developed, it was not until 2012 that an international consensus was unequivocal: after a suspected sport-related concussion, under no circumstances may an athlete return to play on the same day.

It is sometimes assumed that concussion only happens in contact/collision sports such as football and ice hockey. However, concussion may develop in any sport where contact with another athlete or a fall may occur. Indeed, at the National Collegiate Athletic Association (NCAA) level, the concussion rate is highest in men's wrestling, followed by men's and women's ice hockey. Women's soccer, women's basketball, and women's lacrosse have concussion rates similar to men's football. Thus, there should be a low threshold for suspecting concussion when an athlete has been injured and is displaying any of the common symptoms of concussion.

The most commonly used sideline assessment tool is the Sport Concussion Assessment Tool-5 (see Appendix 1 for SCAT5 and Appendix 2 for Child SCAT5). This tool has been validated and provides a broad overview of how to manage suspected sport-related concussion on the sideline. As with any suspected head injury, the clinician should first assess for the possibility of cervical spine injury, skull fracture, or more severe intracranial injury. If the athlete is unconscious, he or she should be managed as if one of these more severe injuries has occurred. Possible "red flag" concerns should be considered in the initial evaluation. (Box 2.1)

In youth sports, it is common that a clinician such as an athletic trainer or physician is not present at the sideline. In these circumstances, it is important for officials, coaches, and parents to be ready to intervene if there is a suspected concussion. The Concussion Recognition Tool 5 (Appendix 3) was developed to help non-clinicians identify athletes with a suspected concussion. This tool outlines "red flags" that should trigger immediate activation of Emergency Medical Services, and also provides common-sense guidance for removal from play for any suspected concussion. Importantly, these athletes must be assessed medically before being allowed to return to play or competition.

If an athlete is injured and concussion is suspected, providers should look for the following signs: movement abnormalities, including lack of movement or uncoordinated, stumbling movements; a vacant look; facial injury; disorientation; and inability to respond to basic questions of orientation. For any suspected sport-related concussion, it is best to evaluate the patient in a quiet place away from the field of play, although this may not always be possible.

If a concussion is suspected—even if it is not clinically confirmed—the athlete must not be allowed to return to play that same day. Importantly, concussion is a process and not a singular event; an athlete's symptoms may evolve over minutes, hours, or even several days. Thus, all athletes with a suspected concussion should be observed serially. The athlete and another responsible adult should receive instructions for the recovery period, which include referral to the Emergency Department if the athlete's condition progressively deteriorates. Importantly, follow-up with a physician/sport clinician should be arranged within days to help assure a proper and graduated return to activity.

TAKE-HOME POINTS

- Concussion may develop in any sport where contact or falls occur.
- More serious injury and "red flags" should always be considered following sport-related concussion.
- No athlete may return to play on the same day as a suspected concussion.
- Serial evaluations of concussion should occur.
- Instructions and prompt referral for follow-up should be normalized.

APPENDIX 2.1: THE SCAT5

BJSM Online First, published on April 26, 2017 as 10.1136/bjsports-2017-097506SCAT5

To download a clean version of the SCAT tools please visit the journal online (http://dx.doi.org/10.1136/bjsports-2017-097506SCAT5)

SCAT5®

SPORT CONCUSSION ASSESSMENT TOOL – 5TH EDITION
DEVELOPED BY THE CONCUSSION IN SPORT GROUP
FOR USE BY MEDICAL PROFESSIONALS ONLY

supported by

 FIFA° 🎗 ⚡ f∃I

Patient details

Name: _____

DOB: _____

Address: _____

ID number: _____

Examiner: _____

Date of Injury: _____ Time: _____

WHAT IS THE SCAT5?

The SCAT5 is a standardized tool for evaluating concussions designed for use by physicians and licensed healthcare professionals[1]. The SCAT5 cannot be performed correctly in less than 10 minutes.

If you are not a physician or licensed healthcare professional, please use the Concussion Recognition Tool 5 (CRT5). The SCAT5 is to be used for evaluating athletes aged 13 years and older. For children aged 12 years or younger, please use the Child SCAT5.

Preseason SCAT5 baseline testing can be useful for interpreting post-injury test scores, but is not required for that purpose. Detailed instructions for use of the SCAT5 are provided on page 7. Please read through these instructions carefully before testing the athlete. Brief verbal instructions for each test are given in italics. The only equipment required for the tester is a watch or timer.

This tool may be freely copied in its current form for distribution to individuals, teams, groups and organizations. It should not be altered in any way, re-branded or sold for commercial gain. Any revision, translation or reproduction in a digital form requires specific approval by the Concussion in Sport Group.

Recognise and Remove

A head impact by either a direct blow or indirect transmission of force can be associated with a serious and potentially fatal brain injury. If there are significant concerns, including any of the red flags listed in Box 1, then activation of emergency procedures and urgent transport to the nearest hospital should be arranged.

Key points

- Any athlete with suspected concussion should be REMOVED FROM PLAY, medically assessed and monitored for deterioration. No athlete diagnosed with concussion should be returned to play on the day of injury.

- If an athlete is suspected of having a concussion and medical personnel are not immediately available, the athlete should be referred to a medical facility for urgent assessment.

- Athletes with suspected concussion should not drink alcohol, use recreational drugs and should not drive a motor vehicle until cleared to do so by a medical professional.

- Concussion signs and symptoms evolve over time and it is important to consider repeat evaluation in the assessment of concussion.

- The diagnosis of a concussion is a clinical judgment, made by a medical professional. The SCAT5 should NOT be used by itself to make, or exclude, the diagnosis of concussion. An athlete may have a concussion even if their SCAT5 is "normal".

Remember:

- The basic principles of first aid (danger, response, airway, breathing, circulation) should be followed.

- Do not attempt to move the athlete (other than that required for airway management) unless trained to do so.

- Assessment for a spinal cord injury is a critical part of the initial on-field assessment.

- Do not remove a helmet or any other equipment unless trained to do so safely.

© Concussion in Sport Group 2017
Davis GA, et al. Br J Sports Med 2017;0:1–8. doi:10.1136/bjsports-2017-097506SCAT5

1

IMMEDIATE OR ON-FIELD ASSESSMENT

The following elements should be assessed for all athletes who are suspected of having a concussion prior to proceeding to the neurocognitive assessment and ideally should be done on-field after the first first aid / emergency care priorities are completed.

If any of the "Red Flags" or observable signs are noted after a direct or indirect blow to the head, the athlete should be immediately and safely removed from participation and evaluated by a physician or licensed healthcare professional.

Consideration of transportation to a medical facility should be at the discretion of the physician or licensed healthcare professional.

The GCS is important as a standard measure for all patients and can be done serially if necessary in the event of deterioration in conscious state. The Maddocks questions and cervical spine exam are critical steps of the immediate assessment; however, these do not need to be done serially.

Name:	
DOB:	
Address:	
ID number:	
Examiner:	
Date:	

STEP 1: RED FLAGS

RED FLAGS:

- **Neck pain or tenderness**
- **Double vision**
- **Weakness or tingling/ burning in arms or legs**
- **Severe or increasing headache**
- **Seizure or convulsion**
- **Loss of consciousness**
- **Deteriorating conscious state**
- **Vomiting**
- **Increasingly restless, agitated or combative**

STEP 2: OBSERVABLE SIGNS

Witnessed ☐   Observed on Video ☐

Lying motionless on the playing surface	Y	N
Balance / gait difficulties / motor incoordination: stumbling, slow / laboured movements	Y	N
Disorientation or confusion, or an inability to respond appropriately to questions	Y	N
Blank or vacant look	Y	N
Facial injury after head trauma	Y	N

STEP 3: MEMORY ASSESSMENT
MADDOCKS QUESTIONS[2]

"I am going to ask you a few questions, please listen carefully and give your best effort. First, tell me what happened?"

Mark Y for correct answer / N for incorrect

What venue are we at today?	Y	N
Which half is it now?	Y	N
Who scored last in this match?	Y	N
What team did you play last week / game?	Y	N
Did your team win the last game?	Y	N

Note: Appropriate sport-specific questions may be substituted.

STEP 4: EXAMINATION
GLASGOW COMA SCALE (GCS)[3]

Time of assessment			
Date of assessment			
Best eye response (E)			
No eye opening	1	1	1
Eye opening in response to pain	2	2	2
Eye opening to speech	3	3	3
Eyes opening spontaneously	4	4	4
Best verbal response (V)			
No verbal response	1	1	1
Incomprehensible sounds	2	2	2
Inappropriate words	3	3	3
Confused	4	4	4
Oriented	5	5	5
Best motor response (M)			
No motor response	1	1	1
Extension to pain	2	2	2
Abnormal flexion to pain	3	3	3
Flexion / Withdrawal to pain	4	4	4
Localizes to pain	5	5	5
Obeys commands	6	6	6
Glasgow Coma score (E + V + M)			

CERVICAL SPINE ASSESSMENT

Does the athlete report that their neck is pain free at rest?	Y	N
If there is NO neck pain at rest, does the athlete have a full range of ACTIVE pain free movement?	Y	N
Is the limb strength and sensation normal?	Y	N

In a patient who is not lucid or fully conscious, a cervical spine injury should be assumed until proven otherwise.

© Concussion in Sport Group 2017

Davis GA, et al. Br J Sports Med 2017;0:1–8. doi:10.1136/bjsports-2017-097506SCAT5

2

OFFICE OR OFF-FIELD ASSESSMENT

Please note that the neurocognitive assessment should be done in a distraction-free environment with the athlete in a resting state.

STEP 1: ATHLETE BACKGROUND

Sport / team / school: _____

Date / time of injury: _____

Years of education completed: _____

Age: _____

Gender: M / F / Other

Dominant hand: left / neither / right

How many diagnosed concussions has the
athlete had in the past?: _____

When was the most recent concussion?: _____

How long was the recovery (time to being cleared to play)
from the most recent concussion?: _____ (days)

Has the athlete ever been:

Hospitalized for a head injury?	Yes	No
Diagnosed / treated for headache disorder or migraines?	Yes	No
Diagnosed with a learning disability / dyslexia?	Yes	No
Diagnosed with ADD / ADHD?	Yes	No
Diagnosed with depression, anxiety or other psychiatric disorder?	Yes	No

Current medications? If yes, please list:

_____

_____

_____

_____

_____

_____

Name: _____

DOB: _____

Address: _____

ID number: _____

Examiner: _____

Date: _____

2

STEP 2: SYMPTOM EVALUATION

The athlete should be given the symptom form and asked to read this instruction paragraph out loud then complete the symptom scale. For the baseline assessment, the athlete should rate his/her symptoms based on how he/she typically feels and for the post injury assessment the athlete should rate their symptoms at this point in time.

Please Check: ☐ **Baseline** ☐ **Post-injury**

Please hand the form to the athlete

	none	mild		moderate		severe	
Headache	0	1	2	3	4	5	6
"Pressure in head"	0	1	2	3	4	5	6
Neck Pain	0	1	2	3	4	5	6
Nausea or vomiting	0	1	2	3	4	5	6
Dizziness	0	1	2	3	4	5	6
Blurred vision	0	1	2	3	4	5	6
Balance problems	0	1	2	3	4	5	6
Sensitivity to light	0	1	2	3	4	5	6
Sensitivity to noise	0	1	2	3	4	5	6
Feeling slowed down	0	1	2	3	4	5	6
Feeling like "in a fog"	0	1	2	3	4	5	6
"Don't feel right"	0	1	2	3	4	5	6
Difficulty concentrating	0	1	2	3	4	5	6
Difficulty remembering	0	1	2	3	4	5	6
Fatigue or low energy	0	1	2	3	4	5	6
Confusion	0	1	2	3	4	5	6
Drowsiness	0	1	2	3	4	5	6
More emotional	0	1	2	3	4	5	6
Irritability	0	1	2	3	4	5	6
Sadness	0	1	2	3	4	5	6
Nervous or Anxious	0	1	2	3	4	5	6
Trouble falling asleep (if applicable)	0	1	2	3	4	5	6

Total number of symptoms: of 22

Symptom severity score: of 132

Do your symptoms get worse with physical activity? Y N

Do your symptoms get worse with mental activity? Y N

If 100% is feeling perfectly normal, what
percent of normal do you feel?

If not 100%, why?

_____

_____

_____

Please hand form back to examiner

© Concussion in Sport Group 2017

Davis GA, *et al. Br J Sports Med* 2017;**0**:1–8. doi:10.1136/bjsports-2017-097506SCAT5

3

3

STEP 3: COGNITIVE SCREENING
Standardised Assessment of Concussion (SAC)[4]

ORIENTATION

	0	1
What month is it?	0	1
What is the date today?	0	1
What is the day of the week?	0	1
What year is it?	0	1
What time is it right now? (within 1 hour)	0	1
Orientation score		of 5

Name: _____
DOB: _____
Address: _____
ID number: _____
Examiner: _____
Date: _____

IMMEDIATE MEMORY

The Immediate Memory component can be completed using the traditional 5-word per trial list or optionally using 10-words per trial to minimise any ceiling effect. All 3 trials must be administered irrespective of the number correct on the first trial. Administer at the rate of one word per second.

Please choose EITHER the 5 or 10 word list groups and circle the specific word list chosen for this test.

I am going to test your memory. I will read you a list of words and when I am done, repeat back as many words as you can remember, in any order. For Trials 2 & 3: I am going to repeat the same list again. Repeat back as many words as you can remember in any order, even if you said the word before.

List	Alternate 5 word lists					Score (of 5)		
						Trial 1	Trial 2	Trial 3
A	Finger	Penny	Blanket	Lemon	Insect			
B	Candle	Paper	Sugar	Sandwich	Wagon			
C	Baby	Monkey	Perfume	Sunset	Iron			
D	Elbow	Apple	Carpet	Saddle	Bubble			
E	Jacket	Arrow	Pepper	Cotton	Movie			
F	Dollar	Honey	Mirror	Saddle	Anchor			
				Immediate Memory Score		of 15		
				Time that last trial was completed				

List	Alternate 10 word lists					Score (of 10)		
						Trial 1	Trial 2	Trial 3
G	Finger	Penny	Blanket	Lemon	Insect			
	Candle	Paper	Sugar	Sandwich	Wagon			
H	Baby	Monkey	Perfume	Sunset	Iron			
	Elbow	Apple	Carpet	Saddle	Bubble			
I	Jacket	Arrow	Pepper	Cotton	Movie			
	Dollar	Honey	Mirror	Saddle	Anchor			
				Immediate Memory Score		of 30		
				Time that last trial was completed				

CONCENTRATION

DIGITS BACKWARDS

Please circle the Digit list chosen (A, B, C, D, E, F). Administer at the rate of one digit per second reading DOWN the selected column.

I am going to read a string of numbers and when I am done, you repeat them back to me in reverse order of how I read them to you. For example, if I say 7-1-9, you would say 9-1-7.

Concentration Number Lists (circle one)

List A	List B	List C			
4-9-3	5-2-6	1-4-2	Y	N	0
6-2-9	4-1-5	6-5-8	Y	N	1
3-8-1-4	1-7-9-5	6-8-3-1	Y	N	0
3-2-7-9	4-9-6-8	3-4-8-1	Y	N	1
6-2-9-7-1	4-8-5-2-7	4-9-1-5-3	Y	N	0
1-5-2-8-6	6-1-8-4-3	6-8-2-5-1	Y	N	1
7-1-8-4-6-2	8-3-1-9-6-4	3-7-6-5-1-9	Y	N	0
5-3-9-1-4-8	7-2-4-8-5-6	9-2-6-5-1-4	Y	N	1

List D	List E	List F			
7-8-2	3-8-2	2-7-1	Y	N	0
9-2-6	5-1-8	4-7-9	Y	N	1
4-1-8-3	2-7-9-3	1-6-8-3	Y	N	0
9-7-2-3	2-1-6-9	3-9-2-4	Y	N	1
1-7-9-2-6	4-1-8-6-9	2-4-7-5-8	Y	N	0
4-1-7-5-2	9-4-1-7-5	8-3-9-6-4	Y	N	1
2-5-4-8-1-7	6-9-7-3-8-2	5-8-6-2-4-9	Y	N	0
8-4-1-9-3-5	4-2-7-9-3-8	3-1-7-9-2-6	Y	N	1
		Digits Score:			of 4

MONTHS IN REVERSE ORDER

Now tell me the months of the year in reverse order. Start with the last month and go backward. So you'll say December, November. Go ahead.

Dec - Nov - Oct - Sept - Aug - Jul - Jun - May - Apr - Mar - Feb - Jan   0   1

Months Score	of 1
Concentration Total Score (Digits + Months)	of 5

© Concussion in Sport Group 2017

Davis GA, et al. Br J Sports Med 2017;0:1–8. doi:10.1136/bjsports-2017-097506SCAT5

4

4

STEP 4: NEUROLOGICAL SCREEN

See the instruction sheet (page 7) for details of
test administration and scoring of the tests.

Can the patient read aloud (e.g. symptom check-list) and follow instructions without difficulty?	Y	N
Does the patient have a full range of pain-free PASSIVE cervical spine movement?	Y	N
Without moving their head or neck, can the patient look side-to-side and up-and-down without double vision?	Y	N
Can the patient perform the finger nose coordination test normally?	Y	N
Can the patient perform tandem gait normally?	Y	N

BALANCE EXAMINATION

Modified Balance Error Scoring System (mBESS) testing[5]

Which foot was tested
(i.e. which is the non-dominant foot)   ☐ Left
                                               ☐ Right

Testing surface (hard floor, field, etc.) _____
Footwear (shoes, barefoot, braces, tape, etc.) _____

Condition	Errors
Double leg stance	of 10
Single leg stance (non-dominant foot)	of 10
Tandem stance (non-dominant foot at the back)	of 10
Total Errors	of 30

Name: _____
DOB: _____
Address: _____
ID number: _____
Examiner: _____
Date: _____

5

STEP 5: DELAYED RECALL:

The delayed recall should be performed after 5 minutes have
elapsed since the end of the Immediate Recall section. Score 1
pt. for each correct response.

*Do you remember that list of words I read a few times earlier? Tell me as many words
from the list as you can remember in any order.*

Time Started _____

Please record each word correctly recalled. Total score equals number of words recalled.

_____
_____
_____
_____

Total number of words recalled accurately: of 5   or   of 10

6

STEP 6: DECISION

Domain	Date & time of assessment:		
Symptom number (of 22)			
Symptom severity score (of 132)			
Orientation (of 5)			
Immediate memory	of 15 of 30	of 15 of 30	of 15 of 30
Concentration (of 5)			
Neuro exam	Normal Abnormal	Normal Abnormal	Normal Abnormal
Balance errors (of 90)			
Delayed Recall	of 5 of 10	of 5 of 10	of 5 of 10

Date and time of injury: _____

If the athlete is known to you prior to their injury, are they different from their usual self?
☐ Yes ☐ No ☐ Unsure ☐ Not Applicable
(If different, describe why in the clinical notes section)

Concussion Diagnosed?
☐ Yes ☐ No ☐ Unsure ☐ Not Applicable

If re-testing, has the athlete improved?
☐ Yes ☐ No ☐ Unsure ☐ Not Applicable

I am a physician or licensed healthcare professional and I have personally
administered or supervised the administration of this SCAT5.

Signature: _____
Name: _____
Title: _____
Registration number (if applicable): _____
Date: _____

**SCORING ON THE SCAT5 SHOULD NOT BE USED AS A STAND-ALONE
METHOD TO DIAGNOSE CONCUSSION, MEASURE RECOVERY OR
MAKE DECISIONS ABOUT AN ATHLETE'S READINESS TO RETURN TO
COMPETITION AFTER CONCUSSION.**

© Concussion in Sport Group 2017
Davis GA, et al. Br J Sports Med 2017;**0**:1–8. doi:10.1136/bjsports-2017-097506SCAT5   5

CLINICAL NOTES:

Name: _____
DOB: _____
Address: _____
ID number: _____
Examiner: _____
Date: _____

_____
_____
_____
_____

_____
_____
_____
_____
_____
_____
_____
_____
_____
_____
_____

✂ ·

CONCUSSION INJURY ADVICE

(To be given to the person monitoring the concussed athlete)

This patient has received an injury to the head. A careful medical examination has been carried out and no sign of any serious complications has been found. Recovery time is variable across individuals and the patient will need monitoring for a further period by a responsible adult. Your treating physician will provide guidance as to this timeframe.

If you notice any change in behaviour, vomiting, worsening headache, double vision or excessive drowsiness, please telephone your doctor or the nearest hospital emergency department immediately.

Other important points:

Initial rest: Limit physical activity to routine daily activities (avoid exercise, training, sports) and limit activities such as school, work, and screen time to a level that does not worsen symptoms.

1) Avoid alcohol

2) Avoid prescription or non-prescription drugs without medical supervision. Specifically:

   a) Avoid sleeping tablets

   b) Do not use aspirin, anti-inflammatory medication or stronger pain medications such as narcotics

3) Do not drive until cleared by a healthcare professional.

4) Return to play/sport requires clearance by a healthcare professional.

Clinic phone number: _____

Patient's name: _____

Date / time of injury: _____

Date / time of medical review: _____

Healthcare Provider: _____

© Concussion in Sport Group 2017

Contact details or stamp

Davis GA, et al. Br J Sports Med 2017;0:1–8. doi:10.1136/bjsports-2017-097506SCAT5

6

INSTRUCTIONS

Words in *Italics* throughout the SCAT5 are the instructions given to the athlete by the clinician

Symptom Scale

The time frame for symptoms should be based on the type of test being administered. At baseline it is advantageous to assess how an athlete "typically" feels whereas during the acute/post-acute stage it is best to ask how the athlete feels at the time of testing.

The symptom scale should be completed by the athlete, not by the examiner. In situations where the symptom scale is being completed after exercise, it should be done in a resting state, generally by approximating his/her resting heart rate.

For total number of symptoms, maximum possible is 22 except immediately post injury, if sleep item is omitted, which then creates a maximum of 21.

For Symptom severity score, add all scores in table, maximum possible is 22 x 6 = 132, except immediately post injury if sleep item is omitted, which then creates a maximum of 21x6=126.

Immediate Memory

The Immediate Memory component can be completed using the traditional 5-word per trial list or, optionally, using 10-words per trial. The literature suggests that the Immediate Memory has a notable ceiling effect when a 5-word list is used. In settings where this ceiling is prominent, the examiner may wish to make the task more difficult by incorporating two 5–word groups for a total of 10 words per trial. In this case, the maximum score per trial is 10 with a total trial maximum of 30.

Choose one of the word lists (either 5 or 10). Then perform 3 trials of immediate memory using this list.

Complete all 3 trials regardless of score on previous trials.

I am going to test your memory. I will read you a list of words and when I am done, repeat back as many words as you can remember, in any order. The words must be read at a rate of one word per second.

Trials 2 & 3 MUST be completed regardless of score on trial 1 & 2.

Trials 2 & 3:

I am going to repeat the same list again. Repeat back as many words as you can remember in any order, even if you said the word before.

Score 1 pt. for each correct response. Total score equals sum across all 3 trials. Do NOT inform the athlete that delayed recall will be tested.

Concentration

Digits backward

Choose one column of digits from lists A, B, C, D, E or F and administer those digits as follows:

Say: *"I am going to read a string of numbers and when I am done, you repeat them back to me in reverse order of how I read them to you. For example, if I say 7-1-9, you would say 9-1-7."*

Begin with first 3 digit string.

If correct, circle "Y" for correct and go to next string length. If incorrect, circle "N" for the first string length and read trial 2 in the same string length. One point possible for each string length. Stop after incorrect on both trials (2 N's) in a string length. The digits should be read at the rate of one per second.

Months in reverse order

"Now tell me the months of the year in reverse order. Start with the last month and go backward. So you'll say December, November ... Go ahead"

1 pt. for entire sequence correct

Delayed Recall

The delayed recall should be performed after 5 minutes have elapsed since the end of the Immediate Recall section.

"Do you remember that list of words I read a few times earlier? Tell me as many words from the list as you can remember in any order."

Score 1 pt. for each correct response

Modified Balance Error Scoring System (mBESS)[5] testing

This balance testing is based on a modified version of the Balance Error Scoring System (BESS)[5]. A timing device is required for this testing.

Each of 20-second trial/stance is scored by counting the number of errors. The examiner will begin counting errors only after the athlete has assumed the proper start position. The modified BESS is calculated by adding one point for each error during the three 20-second tests. The maximum number of errors for any single condition is 10. If the athlete commits multiple errors simultaneously, only

one error is recorded but the athlete should quickly return to the testing position, and counting should resume once the athlete is set. Athletes that are unable to maintain the testing procedure for a minimum of five seconds at the start are assigned the highest possible score, ten, for that testing condition.

OPTION: For further assessment, the same 3 stances can be performed on a surface of medium density foam (e.g., approximately 50cm x 40cm x 6cm).

Balance testing – types of errors

1. Hands lifted off iliac crest	3. Step, stumble, or fall	5. Lifting forefoot or heel
2. Opening eyes	4. Moving hip into > 30 degrees abduction	6. Remaining out of test position > 5 sec

"I am now going to test your balance. Please take your shoes off (if applicable), roll up your pant legs above ankle (if applicable), and remove any ankle taping (if applicable). This test will consist of three twenty second tests with different stances."

(a) Double leg stance:

"The first stance is standing with your feet together with your hands on your hips and with your eyes closed. You should try to maintain stability in that position for 20 seconds. I will be counting the number of times you move out of this position. I will start timing when you are set and have closed your eyes."

(b) Single leg stance:

"If you were to kick a ball, which foot would you use? [This will be the dominant foot] *Now stand on your non-dominant foot. The dominant leg should be held in approximately 30 degrees of hip flexion and 45 degrees of knee flexion. Again, you should try to maintain stability for 20 seconds with your hands on your hips and your eyes closed. I will be counting the number of times you move out of this position. If you stumble out of this position, open your eyes and return to the start position and continue balancing. I will start timing when you are set and have closed your eyes."*

(c) Tandem stance:

"Now stand heel-to-toe with your non-dominant foot in back. Your weight should be evenly distributed across both feet. Again, you should try to maintain stability for 20 seconds with your hands on your hips and your eyes closed. I will be counting the number of times you move out of this position. If you stumble out of this position, open your eyes and return to the start position and continue balancing. I will start timing when you are set and have closed your eyes."

Tandem Gait

Participants are instructed to stand with their feet together behind a starting line (the test is best done with footwear removed). Then, they walk in a forward direction as quickly and as accurately as possible along a 38mm wide (sports tape), 3 metre line with an alternate foot heel-to-toe gait ensuring that they approximate their heel and toe on each step. Once they cross the end of the 3m line, they turn 180 degrees and return to the starting point using the same gait. Athletes fail the test if they step off the line, have a separation between their heel and toe, or if they touch or grab the examiner or an object.

Finger to Nose

"I am going to test your coordination now. Please sit comfortably on the chair with your eyes open and your arm (either right or left) outstretched (shoulder flexed to 90 degrees and elbow and fingers extended), pointing in front of you. When I give a start signal, I would like you to perform five successive finger to nose repetitions using your index finger to touch the tip of the nose, and then return to the starting position, as quickly and as accurately as possible."

References

1. McCrory et al. Consensus Statement On Concussion In Sport – The 5th International Conference On Concussion In Sport Held In Berlin, October 2016. British Journal of Sports Medicine 2017 (available at www.bjsm.bmj.com)

2. Maddocks, DL; Dicker, GD; Saling, MM. The assessment of orientation following concussion in athletes. Clinical Journal of Sport Medicine 1995; 5: 32-33

3. Jennett, B., Bond, M. Assessment of outcome after severe brain damage: a practical scale. Lancet 1975; I: 480-484

4. McCrea M. Standardized mental status testing of acute concussion. Clinical Journal of Sport Medicine. 2001; 11: 176-181

5. Guskiewicz KM. Assessment of postural stability following sport-related concussion. Current Sports Medicine Reports. 2003; 2: 24-30

© Concussion in Sport Group 2017

CONCUSSION INFORMATION

Any athlete suspected of having a concussion should be removed from play and seek medical evaluation.

Signs to watch for

Problems could arise over the first 24-48 hours. The athlete should not be left alone and must go to a hospital at once if they experience:

- Worsening headache
- Repeated vomiting
- Weakness or numbness in arms or legs
- Drowsiness or inability to be awakened
- Unusual behaviour or confusion or irritable
- Unsteadiness on their feet.
- Inability to recognize people or places
- Seizures (arms and legs jerk uncontrollably)
- Slurred speech

Consult your physician or licensed healthcare professional after a suspected concussion. Remember, it is better to be safe.

Rest & Rehabilitation

After a concussion, the athlete should have physical rest and relative cognitive rest for a few days to allow their symptoms to improve. In most cases, after no more than a few days of rest, the athlete should gradually increase their daily activity level as long as their symptoms do not worsen. Once the athlete is able to complete their usual daily activities without concussion-related symptoms, the second step of the return to play/sport progression can be started. The athlete should not return to play/sport until their concussion-related symptoms have resolved and the athlete has successfully returned to full school/learning activities.

When returning to play/sport, the athlete should follow a stepwise, medically managed exercise progression, with increasing amounts of exercise. For example:

Graduated Return to Sport Strategy

Exercise step	Functional exercise at each step	Goal of each step
1. Symptom-limited activity	Daily activities that do not provoke symptoms.	Gradual reintroduction of work/school activities.
2. Light aerobic exercise	Walking or stationary cycling at slow to medium pace. No resistance training.	Increase heart rate.
3. Sport-specific exercise	Running or skating drills. No head impact activities.	Add movement.
4. Non-contact training drills	Harder training drills, e.g., passing drills. May start progressive resistance training.	Exercise, coordination, and increased thinking.
5. Full contact practice	Following medical clearance, participate in normal training activities.	Restore confidence and assess functional skills by coaching staff.
6. Return to play/sport	Normal game play.	

In this example, it would be typical to have 24 hours (or longer) for each step of the progression. If any symptoms worsen while exercising, the athlete should go back to the previous step. Resistance training should be added only in the later stages (Stage 3 or 4 at the earliest).

Written clearance should be provided by a healthcare professional before return to play/sport as directed by local laws and regulations.

Graduated Return to School Strategy

Concussion may affect the ability to learn at school. The athlete may need to miss a few days of school after a concussion. When going back to school, some athletes may need to go back gradually and may need to have some changes made to their schedule so that concussion symptoms do not get worse. If a particular activity makes symptoms worse, then the athlete should stop that activity and rest until symptoms get better. To make sure that the athlete can get back to school without problems, it is important that the healthcare provider, parents, caregivers and teachers talk to each other so that everyone knows what the plan is for the athlete to go back to school.

Note: If mental activity does not cause any symptoms, the athlete may be able to skip step 2 and return to school part-time before doing school activities at home first.

Mental Activity	Activity at each step	Goal of each step
1. Daily activities that do not give the athlete symptoms	Typical activities that the athlete does during the day as long as they do not increase symptoms (e.g. reading, texting, screen time). Start with 5-15 minutes at a time and gradually build up.	Gradual return to typical activities.
2. School activities	Homework, reading or other cognitive activities outside of the classroom.	Increase tolerance to cognitive work.
3. Return to school part-time	Gradual introduction of school-work. May need to start with a partial school day or with increased breaks during the day.	Increase academic activities.
4. Return to school full-time	Gradually progress school activities until a full day can be tolerated.	Return to full academic activities and catch up on missed work.

If the athlete continues to have symptoms with mental activity, some other accomodations that can help with return to school may include:

- Starting school later, only going for half days, or going only to certain classes
- More time to finish assignments/tests
- Quiet room to finish assignments/tests
- Not going to noisy areas like the cafeteria, assembly halls, sporting events, music class, shop class, etc.
- Taking lots of breaks during class, homework, tests
- No more than one exam/day
- Shorter assignments
- Repetition/memory cues
- Use of a student helper/tutor
- Reassurance from teachers that the child will be supported while getting better

The athlete should not go back to sports until they are back to school/learning, without symptoms getting significantly worse and no longer needing any changes to their schedule.

Davis GA, et al. Br J Sports Med 2017;0:1–8. doi:10.1136/bjsports-2017-097506SCAT5

8

APPENDIX 2.2: THE CHILD SCAT5

BJSM Online First, published on April 28, 2017 as 10.1136/bjsports-2017-097492childscat5

Child SCAT5®

SPORT CONCUSSION ASSESSMENT TOOL
FOR CHILDREN AGES 5 TO 12 YEARS
FOR USE BY MEDICAL PROFESSIONALS ONLY

supported by

Patient details

Name: _____

DOB: _____

Address: _____

ID number: _____

Examiner: _____

Date of Injury: _____ Time: _____

WHAT IS THE CHILD SCAT5?

The Child SCAT5 is a standardized tool for evaluating concussions designed for use by physicians and licensed healthcare professionals[1].

If you are not a physician or licensed healthcare professional, please use the Concussion Recognition Tool 5 (CRT5). The Child SCAT5 is to be used for evaluating Children aged 5 to 12 years. For athletes aged 13 years and older, please use the SCAT5.

Preseason Child SCAT5 baseline testing can be useful for interpreting post-injury test scores, but not required for that purpose. Detailed instructions for use of the Child SCAT5 are provided on page 7. Please read through these instructions carefully before testing the athlete. Brief verbal instructions for each test are given in italics. The only equipment required for the tester is a watch or timer.

This tool may be freely copied in its current form for distribution to individuals, teams, groups and organizations. It should not be altered in any way, re-branded or sold for commercial gain. Any revision, translation or reproduction in a digital form requires specific approval by the Concussion in Sport Group.

Recognise and Remove

A head impact by either a direct blow or indirect transmission of force can be associated with a serious and potentially fatal brain injury. If there are significant concerns, including any of the red flags listed in Box 1, then activation of emergency procedures and urgent transport to the nearest hospital should be arranged.

Key points

- Any athlete with suspected concussion should be REMOVED FROM PLAY, medically assessed and monitored for deterioration. No athlete diagnosed with concussion should be returned to play on the day of injury.

- If the child is suspected of having a concussion and medical personnel are not immediately available, the child should be referred to a medical facility for urgent assessment.

- Concussion signs and symptoms evolve over time and it is important to consider repeat evaluation in the assessment of concussion.

- The diagnosis of a concussion is a clinical judgment, made by a medical professional. The Child SCAT5 should NOT be used by itself to make, or exclude, the diagnosis of concussion. An athlete may have a a concussion even if their Child SCAT5 is "normal".

Remember:

- The basic principles of first aid (danger, response, airway, breathing, circulation) should be followed.

- Do not attempt to move the athlete (other than that required for airway management) unless trained to do so.

- Assessment for a spinal cord injury is a critical part of the initial on-field assessment.

- Do not remove a helmet or any other equipment unless trained to do so safely.

1

1

IMMEDIATE OR ON-FIELD ASSESSMENT

The following elements should be assessed for all athletes who are suspected of having a concussion prior to proceeding to the neurocognitive assessment and ideally should be done on-field after the first first aid / emergency care priorities are completed.

If any of the "Red Flags" or observable signs are noted after a direct or indirect blow to the head, the athlete should be immediately and safely removed from participation and evaluated by a physician or licensed healthcare professional.

Consideration of transportation to a medical facility should be at the discretion of the physician or licensed healthcare professional.

The GCS is important as a standard measure for all patients and can be done serially if necessary in the event of deterioration in conscious state. The cervical spine exam is a critical step of the immediate assessment, however, it does not need to be done serially.

STEP 1: RED FLAGS

RED FLAGS:	
• Neck pain or tenderness	• Seizure or convulsion
• Double vision	• Loss of consciousness
• Weakness or tingling/ burning in arms or legs	• Deteriorating conscious state
• Severe or increasing headache	• Vomiting
	• Increasingly restless, agitated or combative

STEP 2: OBSERVABLE SIGNS

Witnessed ☐   Observed on Video ☐

Lying motionless on the playing surface	Y	N
Balance / gait difficulties / motor incoordination: stumbling, slow / laboured movements	Y	N
Disorientation or confusion, or an inability to respond appropriately to questions	Y	N
Blank or vacant look	Y	N
Facial injury after head trauma	Y	N

STEP 3: EXAMINATION
GLASGOW COMA SCALE (GCS)[2]

Time of assessment			
Date of assessment			
Best eye response (E)			
No eye opening	1	1	1
Eye opening in response to pain	2	2	2
Eye opening to speech	3	3	3
Eyes opening spontaneously	4	4	4
Best verbal response (V)			
No verbal response	1	1	1

Name: _____
DOB: _____
Address: _____
ID number: _____
Examiner: _____
Date: _____

Incomprehensible sounds	2	2	2
Inappropriate words	3	3	3
Confused	4	4	4
Oriented	5	5	5
Best motor response (M)			
No motor response	1	1	1
Extension to pain	2	2	2
Abnormal flexion to pain	3	3	3
Flexion / Withdrawal to pain	4	4	4
Localizes to pain	5	5	5
Obeys commands	6	6	6
Glasgow Coma score (E + V + M)			

CERVICAL SPINE ASSESSMENT

Does the athlete report that their neck is pain free at rest?	Y	N
If there is NO neck pain at rest, does the athlete have a full range of ACTIVE pain free movement?	Y	N
Is the limb strength and sensation normal?	Y	N

In a patient who is not lucid or fully conscious, a cervical spine injury should be assumed until proven otherwise.

OFFICE OR OFF-FIELD ASSESSMENT
STEP 1: ATHLETE BACKGROUND

Please note that the neurocognitive assessment should be done in a distraction-free environment with the athlete in a resting state.

Sport / team / school: _____
Date / time of injury: _____
Years of education completed: _____
Age: _____
Gender: M / F / Other
Dominant hand: left / neither / right
How many diagnosed concussions has the athlete had in the past?: _____
When was the most recent concussion?: _____
How long was the recovery (time to being cleared to play) from the most recent concussion?: _____ (days)

Has the athlete ever been:

Hospitalized for a head injury?	Yes	No
Diagnosed / treated for headache disorder or migraines?	Yes	No
Diagnosed with a learning disability / dyslexia?	Yes	No
Diagnosed with ADD / ADHD?	Yes	No
Diagnosed with depression, anxiety or other psychiatric disorder?	Yes	No

Current medications? If yes, please list: _____

© Concussion in Sport Group 2017

2

STEP 2: SYMPTOM EVALUATION

The athlete should be given the symptom form and asked to read this instruction paragraph out loud then complete the symptom scale. For the baseline assessment, the athlete should rate his/her symptoms based on how he/she typically feels and for the post injury assessment the athlete should rate their symptoms at this point in time.

To be done in a resting state

Please Check: ☐ Baseline ☐ Post-Injury

Name: _____
DOB: _____
Address: _____
ID number: _____
Examiner: _____
Date: _____

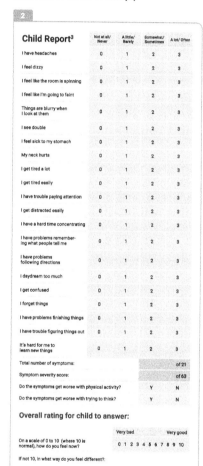

Child Report[3]

	Not at all/ Never	A little/ Rarely	Somewhat/ Sometimes	A lot/ Often
I have headaches	0	1	2	3
I feel dizzy	0	1	2	3
I feel like the room is spinning	0	1	2	3
I feel like I'm going to faint	0	1	2	3
Things are blurry when I look at them	0	1	2	3
I see double	0	1	2	3
I feel sick to my stomach	0	1	2	3
My neck hurts	0	1	2	3
I get tired a lot	0	1	2	3
I get tired easily	0	1	2	3
I have trouble paying attention	0	1	2	3
I get distracted easily	0	1	2	3
I have a hard time concentrating	0	1	2	3
I have problems remembering what people tell me	0	1	2	3
I have problems following directions	0	1	2	3
I daydream too much	0	1	2	3
I get confused	0	1	2	3
I forget things	0	1	2	3
I have problems finishing things	0	1	2	3
I have trouble figuring things out	0	1	2	3
It's hard for me to learn new things	0	1	2	3
Total number of symptoms:				of 21
Symptom severity score:				of 63
Do the symptoms get worse with physical activity?			Y	N
Do the symptoms get worse with trying to think?			Y	N

Overall rating for child to answer:

	Very bad		Very good
On a scale of 0 to 10 (where 10 is normal), how do you feel now?	0 1 2 3 4 5 6 7 8 9 10		

If not 10, in what way do you feel different?:

Parent Report

The child:

	Not at all/ Never	A little/ Rarely	Somewhat/ Sometimes	A lot/ Often
has headaches	0	1	2	3
feels dizzy	0	1	2	3
has a feeling that the room is spinning	0	1	2	3
feels faint	0	1	2	3
has blurred vision	0	1	2	3
has double vision	0	1	2	3
experiences nausea	0	1	2	3
has a sore neck	0	1	2	3
gets tired a lot	0	1	2	3
gets tired easily	0	1	2	3
has trouble sustaining attention	0	1	2	3
is easily distracted	0	1	2	3
has difficulty concentrating	0	1	2	3
has problems remembering what he/she is told	0	1	2	3
has difficulty following directions	0	1	2	3
tends to daydream	0	1	2	3
gets confused	0	1	2	3
is forgetful	0	1	2	3
has difficulty completing tasks	0	1	2	3
has poor problem solving skills	0	1	2	3
has problems learning	0	1	2	3
Total number of symptoms:				of 21
Symptom severity score:				of 63
Do the symptoms get worse with physical activity?			Y	N
Do the symptoms get worse with mental activity?			Y	N

Overall rating for parent/teacher/coach/carer to answer

On a scale of 0 to 100% (where 100% is normal), how would you rate the child now?

If not 100%, in what way does the child seem different?

© Concussion in Sport Group 2017

3

3

STEP 3: COGNITIVE SCREENING
Standardized Assessment of Concussion - Child Version (SAC-C)[4]

IMMEDIATE MEMORY

The Immediate Memory component can be completed using the traditional 5-word per trial list or optionally using 10-words per trial to minimise any ceiling effect. All 3 trials must be administered irrespective of the number correct on the first trial. Administer at the rate of one word per second.

Please choose EITHER the 5 or 10 word list groups and circle the specific word list chosen for this test.

I am going to test your memory. I will read you a list of words and when I am done, repeat back as many words as you can remember, in any order. For Trials 2 & 3: I am going to repeat the same list again. Repeat back as many words as you can remember in any order, even if you said the word before.

List	Alternate 5 word lists					Score (of 5) Trial 1	Trial 2	Trial 3
A	Finger	Penny	Blanket	Lemon	Insect			
B	Candle	Paper	Sugar	Sandwich	Wagon			
C	Baby	Monkey	Perfume	Sunset	Iron			
D	Elbow	Apple	Carpet	Saddle	Bubble			
E	Jacket	Arrow	Pepper	Cotton	Movie			
F	Dollar	Honey	Mirror	Saddle	Anchor			
				Immediate Memory Score				of 15
				Time that last trial was completed				

List	Alternate 10 word lists					Score (of 10) Trial 1	Trial 2	Trial 3
G	Finger	Penny	Blanket	Lemon	Insect			
	Candle	Paper	Sugar	Sandwich	Wagon			
H	Baby	Monkey	Perfume	Sunset	Iron			
	Elbow	Apple	Carpet	Saddle	Bubble			
I	Jacket	Arrow	Pepper	Cotton	Movie			
	Dollar	Honey	Mirror	Saddle	Anchor			
				Immediate Memory Score				of 30
				Time that last trial was completed				

CONCENTRATION

DIGITS BACKWARDS

Please circle the Digit list chosen (A, B, C, D, E, F). Administer at the rate of one digit per second reading DOWN the selected column.

I am going to read a string of numbers and when I am done, you repeat them back to me in reverse order of how I read them to you. For example, if I say 7-1-9, you would say 9-1-7.

Concentration Number Lists (circle one)

List A	List B	List C			
5-2	4-1	4-9	Y	N	0
4-1	9-4	6-2	Y	N	1
4-9-3	5-2-6	1-4-2	Y	N	0
6-2-9	4-1-5	6-5-8	Y	N	1
3-8-1-4	1-7-9-5	6-8-3-1	Y	N	0
3-2-7-9	4-9-6-8	3-4-8-1	Y	N	1
6-2-9-7-1	4-8-5-2-7	4-9-1-5-3	Y	N	0
1-5-2-8-6	6-1-8-4-3	6-8-2-5-1	Y	N	1
7-1-8-4-6-2	8-3-1-9-6-4	3-7-6-5-1-9	Y	N	0
5-3-9-1-4-8	7-2-4-8-5-5	9-2-6-5-1-4	Y	N	1

List D	List E	List F			
2-7	9-2	7-8	Y	N	0
5-9	6-1	5-1	Y	N	1
7-8-2	3-8-2	2-7-1	Y	N	0
9-2-6	5-1-8	4-7-9	Y	N	1
4-1-8-3	2-7-9-3	1-5-8-3	Y	N	0
9-7-2-3	2-1-6-9-	3-9-2-4	Y	N	1
1-7-9-2-6	4-1-8-6-9	2-4-7-5-8	Y	N	0
4-1-7-5-2	9-4-1-7-5	8-3-9-6-4	Y	N	1
2-6-4-8-1-7	6-9-7-3-8-2	5-8-6-2-4-9	Y	N	0
8-4-1-9-3-5	4-2-7-3-9-8	3-1-7-8-2-6	Y	N	1
		Digits Score:			of 5

DAYS IN REVERSE ORDER

Now tell me the days of the week in reverse order. Start with the last day and go backward. So you'll say Sunday, Saturday. Go ahead.

Sunday - Saturday - Friday - Thursday - Wednesday - Tuesday - Monday	0 1
Days Score	of 1
Concentration Total Score (Digits + Days)	of 6

4

4

STEP 4: NEUROLOGICAL SCREEN

See the instruction sheet (page 7) for details of test administration and scoring of the tests.

Can the patient read aloud (e.g. symptom check-list) and follow instructions without difficulty?	Y	N
Does the patient have a full range of pain-free PASSIVE cervical spine movement?	Y	N
Without moving their head or neck, can the patient look side-to-side and up-and-down without double vision?	Y	N
Can the patient perform the finger nose coordination test normally?	Y	N
Can the patient perform tandem gait normally?	Y	N

BALANCE EXAMINATION

Modified Balance Error Scoring System (BESS) testing[6]

Which foot was tested (i.e. which is the non-dominant foot)	☐ Left ☐ Right

Testing surface (hard floor, field, etc.) _____
Footwear (shoes, barefoot, braces, tape, etc.) _____

Condition	Errors
Double leg stance	of 10
Single leg stance (non-dominant foot, 10-12 y/o only)	of 10
Tandem stance (non-dominant foot at back)	of 10
Total Errors	5-9 y/o of 20 10-12 y/o of 30

Name: _____
DOB: _____
Address: _____
ID number: _____
Examiner: _____
Date: _____

5

STEP 5: DELAYED RECALL:

The delayed recall should be performed after 5 minutes have elapsed since the end of the Immediate Recall section. Score 1 pt. for each correct response.

Do you remember that list of words I read a few times earlier? Tell me as many words from the list as you can remember in any order.

Time Started

Please record each word correctly recalled. Total score equals number of words recalled.

_____
_____
_____
_____

Total number of words recalled accurately:	of 5	or	of 10

6

STEP 6: DECISION

Domain	Date & time of assessment:		
Symptom number Child report (of 21) Parent report (of 21)			
Symptom severity score Child report (of 63) Parent report (of 63)			
Immediate memory	of 15 of 30	of 15 of 30	of 15 of 30
Concentration (of 6)			
Neuro exam	Normal Abnormal	Normal Abnormal	Normal Abnormal
Balance errors (5-9 y/o of 20) (10-12 y/o of 30)			
Delayed Recall	of 5 of 10	of 5 of 10	of 5 of 10

Date and time of injury: _____

If the athlete is known to you prior to their injury, are they different from their usual self?
☐ Yes ☐ No ☐ Unsure ☐ Not Applicable
(If different, describe why in the clinical notes section)

Concussion Diagnosed?
☐ Yes ☐ No ☐ Unsure ☐ Not Applicable

If re-testing, has the athlete improved?
☐ Yes ☐ No ☐ Unsure ☐ Not Applicable

I am a physician or licensed healthcare professional and I have personally administered or supervised the administration of this Child SCAT5.

Signature: _____
Name: _____
Title: _____
Registration number (if applicable): _____
Date: _____

SCORING ON THE CHILD SCAT5 SHOULD NOT BE USED AS A STAND-ALONE METHOD TO DIAGNOSE CONCUSSION, MEASURE RECOVERY OR MAKE DECISIONS ABOUT AN ATHLETE'S READINESS TO RETURN TO COMPETITION AFTER CONCUSSION.

© Concussion in Sport Group 2017

5

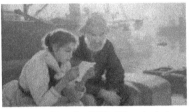

| Name: |
| DOB: |
| Address: |
| ID number: |
| Examiner: |
| Date: |

For the Neurological Screen (page 5), if the child cannot read, ask him/her to describe what they see in this picture.

CLINICAL NOTES:

_____

_____

_____

_____

_____

_____

✂ ·

Concussion injury advice for the child and parents/carergivers

(To be given to the person monitoring the concussed child)

This child has had an injury to the head and needs to be carefully watched for the next 24 hours by a responsible adult.

If you notice any change in behavior, vomiting, dizziness, worsening headache, double vision or excessive drowsiness, please call an ambulance to take the child to hospital immediately.

Other important points:

Following concussion, the child should rest for at least 24 hours.

· The child should not use a computer, internet or play video games if these activities make symptoms worse.

· The child should not be given any medications, including pain killers, unless prescribed by a medical doctor.

· The child should not go back to school until symptoms are improving.

· The child should not go back to sport or play until a doctor gives permission.

Clinic phone number: _____

Patient's name: _____

Date / time of injury: _____

Date / time of medical review: _____

Healthcare Provider: _____

© Concussion in Sport Group 2017

Contact details or stamp

6

INSTRUCTIONS

Words in *Italics* throughout the Child SCAT5 are the instructions given to the athlete by the clinician

Symptom Scale

In situations where the symptom scale is being completed after exercise, it should still be done in a resting state, at least 10 minutes post exercise.

At Baseline	On the day of injury	On all subsequent days
• The child is to complete the Child Report, according to how he/she feels today, and	• The child is to complete the Child Report, according to how he/she feels now.	• The child is to complete the Child Report, according to how she feels today, and
• The parent/carer is to complete the Parent Report according to how the child has been over the previous week.	• If the parent is present, and has had time to assess the child on the day of injury, the parent completes the Parent Report according to how the child appears now.	• The parent/carer is to complete the Parent Report according to how the child has been over the previous 24 hours.

For Total number of symptoms, maximum possible is 21

For Symptom severity score, add all scores in table, maximum possible is 21 x 3 = 63

Standardized Assessment of Concussion Child Version (SAC-C)

Immediate Memory

Choose one of the 5-word lists. Then perform 3 trials of immediate memory using this list.

Complete all 3 trials regardless of score on previous trials.

"I am going to test your memory. I will read you a list of words and when I am done, repeat back as many words as you can remember, in any order." The words must be read at a rate of one word per second.

OPTION: The literature suggests that the Immediate Memory has a notable ceiling effect when a 5-word list is used. (In younger children, use the 5-word list). In settings where this ceiling is prominent the examiner may wish to make the task more difficult by incorporating two 5-word groups for a total of 10 words per trial. In this case the maximum score per trial is 10 with a total trial maximum of 30.

Trials 2 & 3 MUST be completed regardless of score on trial 1 & 2.

Trials 2 & 3: *"I am going to repeat the same list again. Repeat back as many words as you can remember in any order, even if you said the word before."*

Score 1 pt. for each correct response. Total score equals sum across all 3 trials. Do NOT inform the athlete that delayed recall will be tested.

Concentration

Digits backward

Choose one column only, from List A, B, C, D, E or F, and administer those digits as follows:

"I am going to read you some numbers and when I am done, you say them back to me backwards, in reverse order of how I read them to you. For example, if I say 7-1, you would say 1-7."

If correct, circle "Y" for correct and go to next string length. If incorrect, circle "N" for the first string length and read trial 2 in the same string length. One point possible for each string length. Stop after incorrect on both trials (2 N's) in a string length. The digits should be read at the rate of one per second.

Days of the week in reverse order

"Now tell me the days of the week in reverse order. Start with Sunday and go backward. So you'll say Sunday, Saturday ... Go ahead"

1 pt. for entire sequence correct

Delayed Recall

The delayed recall should be performed after at least 5 minutes have elapsed since the end of the Immediate Recall section.

"Do you remember that list of words I read a few times earlier? Tell me as many words from the list as you can remember in any order."

Circle each word correctly recalled. Total score equals number of words recalled.

Neurological Screen

Reading

The child is asked to read a paragraph of text from the instructions in the Child SCAT5. For children who can not read, they are asked to describe what they see in a photograph or picture, such as that on page 6 of the Child SCAT5.

Modified Balance Error Scoring System (mBESS)[5] testing

These instructions are to be read by the person administering the Child SCAT5, and each balance task should be demonstrated to the child. The child should then be asked to copy what the examiner demonstrated.

Each of 20-second trial/stance is scored by counting the number of errors. The This balance testing is based on a modified version of the Balance Error Scoring System (BESS)[1].

A stopwatch or watch with a second hand is required for this testing.

"I am now going to test your balance. Please take your shoes off, roll up your pants above your ankle (if applicable), and remove any ankle taping (if applicable). This test will consist of two different parts."

OPTION: For further assessment, the same 3 stances can be performed on a surface of medium density foam (e.g., approximately 50cm x 40cm x 6cm).

(a) Double leg stance:

The first stance is standing with the feet together with hands on hips and with eyes closed. The child should try to maintain stability in that position for 20 seconds. You should inform the child that you will be counting the number of times the child moves out of this position. You should start timing when the child is set and the eyes are closed.

(b) Tandem stance:

Instruct or show the child how to stand heel-to-toe with the non-dominant foot in the back. Weight should be evenly distributed across both feet. Again, the child should try to maintain stability for 20 seconds with hands on hips and eyes closed. You should inform the child that you will be counting the number of times the child moves out of this position. If the child stumbles out of this position, instruct him/her to open the eyes and return to the start position and continue balancing. You should start timing when the child is set and the eyes are closed.

(c) Single leg stance (10-12 year olds only):

"If you were to kick a ball, which foot would you use? [This will be the dominant foot] Now stand on your other foot. You should bend your other leg and hold it up (show the child). Again, try to stay in that position for 20 seconds with your hands on your hips and your eyes closed. I will be counting the number of times you move out of this position. If you move out of this position, open your eyes and return to the start position and keep balancing. I will start timing once you are set and have closed your eyes."

Balance testing – types of errors

1. Hands lifted off iliac crest	3. Step, stumble, or fall	5. Lifting forefoot or heel
2. Opening eyes	4. Moving hip into > 30 degrees abduction	6. Remaining out of test position > 5 sec

Each of the 20-second trials is scored by counting the errors, or deviations from the proper stance, accumulated by the child. The examiner will begin counting errors only after the child has assumed the proper start position. The modified BESS is calculated by adding one error point for each error during the 20-second trial. The maximum total number of errors for any single condition is 10. If a child commits multiple errors simultaneously, only one error is recorded but the child should quickly return to the testing position, and counting should resume once subject is set. Children who are unable to maintain the testing procedure for a minimum of five seconds at the start are assigned the highest possible score, ten, for that testing condition.

Tandem Gait

Instruction for the examiner - Demonstrate the following to the child:

The child is instructed to stand with their feet together behind a starting line (the test is best done with footwear removed). Then, they walk in a forward direction as quickly and as accurately as possible along a 38mm wide (sports tape), 3 metre line with an alternate foot heel-to-toe gait ensuring that they approximate their heel and toe on each step. Once they cross the end of the 3m line, they turn 180 degrees and return to the starting point using the same gait. Children fail the test if they step off the line, have a separation between their heel and toe, or if they touch or grab the examiner or an object.

Finger to Nose

The tester should demonstrate it to the child.

"I am going to test your coordination now. Please sit comfortably on the chair with your eyes open and your arm (either right or left) outstretched (shoulder flexed to 90 degrees and elbow and fingers extended). When I give a start signal, I would like you to perform five successive finger to nose repetitions using your index finger to touch the tip of the nose as quickly and as accurately as possible."

Scoring: 5 correct repetitions in < 4 seconds = 1

Note for testers: Children fail the test if they do not touch their nose, do not fully extend their elbow or do not perform five repetitions.

References

1. McCrory et al. Consensus Statement On Concussion In Sport – The 5th international Conference On Concussion In Sport Held In Berlin, October 2016. British Journal of Sports Medicine 2017 (available at www.bjsm.bmj.com)

2. Jennett, B., Bond, M. Assessment of outcome after severe brain damage: a practical scale. Lancet 1975; i: 480-484

3. Ayr, L.K., Yeates, K.O., Taylor, H.G., Brown, M. Dimensions of postconcussive symptoms in children with mild traumatic brain injuries. Journal of the International Neuropsychological Society. 2009; 15:19–30

4. McCrea M. Standardized mental status testing of acute concussion. Clinical Journal of Sports Medicine. 2001; 11: 176-181

5. Guskiewicz KM. Assessment of postural stability following sport-related concussion. Current Sports Medicine Reports. 2003; 2: 24-30

© Concussion in Sport Group 2017

7

CONCUSSION INFORMATION

If you think you or a teammate has a concussion, tell your coach/trainer/parent right away so that you can be taken out of the game. You or your teammate should be seen by a doctor as soon as possible. YOU OR YOUR TEAMMATE SHOULD NOT GO BACK TO PLAY/SPORT THAT DAY.

Signs to watch for

Problems can happen over the first 24-48 hours. You or your teammate should not be left alone and must go to a hospital right away if any of the following happens:

- New headache, or headache gets worse
- Neck pain that gets worse
- Becomes sleepy/drowsy or can't be woken up
- Cannot recognise people or places

- Feeling sick to your stomach or vomiting
- Acting weird/strange, seems/feels confused, or is irritable
- Has any seizures (arms and/or legs jerk uncontroliably)

- Has weakness, numbness or tingling (arms, legs or face)
- Is unsteady walking or standing
- Talking is slurred
- Cannot understand what someone is saying or directions

Consult your physician or licensed healthcare professional after a suspected concussion. Remember, it is better to be safe.

Graduated Return to Sport Strategy

After a concussion, the child should rest physically and mentally for a few days to allow symptoms to get better. In most cases, after a few days of rest, they can gradually increase their daily activity level as long as symptoms don't get worse. Once they are able to do their usual daily activities without symptoms, the child should gradually increase exercise in steps, guided by the healthcare professional (see below).

The athlete should not return to play/sport the day of injury.

NOTE: An initial period of a few days of both cognitive ("thinking") and physical rest is recommended before beginning the Return to Sport progression.

Exercise step	Functional exercise at each step	Goal of each step
1. Symptom-limited activity	Daily activities that do not provoke symptoms.	Gradual reintroduction of work/school activities.
2. Light aerobic exercise	Walking or stationary cycling at slow to medium pace. No resistance training.	Increase heart rate.
3. Sport-specific exercise	Running or skating drills. No head impact activities.	Add movement.
4. Non-contact training drills	Harder training drills, e.g., passing drills. May start progressive resistance training.	Exercise, coordination, and increased thinking.
5. Full contact practice	Following medical clearance, participate in normal training activities.	Restore confidence and assess functional skills by coaching staff.
6. Return to play/sport	Normal game play.	

There should be at least 24 hours (or longer) for each step of the progression. If any symptoms worsen while exercising, the athlete should go back to the previous step. Resistance training should be added only in the later stages (Stage 3 or 4 at the earliest). The athlete should not return to sport until the concussion symptoms have gone, they have successfully returned to full school/learning activities, and the healthcare professional has given the child written permission to return to sport.

If the child has symptoms for more than a month, they should ask to be referred to a healthcare professional who is an expert in the management of concussion.

Graduated Return to School Strategy

Concussion may affect the ability to learn at school. The child may need to miss a few days of school after a concussion, but the child's doctor should help them get back to school after a few days. When going back to school, some children may need to go back gradually and may need to have some changes made to their schedule so that concussion symptoms don't get a lot worse. If a particular activity makes symptoms a lot worse, then the child should stop that activity and rest until symptoms get better. To make sure that the child can get back to school without problems, it is important that the health care provider, parents/caregivers and teachers talk to each other so that everyone knows what the plan is for the child to go back to school.

Note: If mental activity does not cause any symptoms, the child may be able to return to school part-time without doing school activities at home first.

Mental Activity	Activity at each step	Goal of each step
1. Daily activities that do not give the child symptoms	Typical activities that the child does during the day as long as they do not increase symptoms (e.g. reading, texting, screen time). Start with 5-15 minutes at a time and gradually build up.	Gradual return to typical activities.
2. School activities	Homework, reading or other cognitive activities outside of the classroom.	Increase tolerance to cognitive work.
3. Return to school part-time	Gradual introduction of schoolwork. May need to start with a partial school day or with increased breaks during the day.	Increase academic activities.
4. Return to school full-time	Gradually progress school activities until a full day can be tolerated.	Return to full academic activities and catch up on missed work.

If the child continues to have symptoms with mental activity, some other things that can be done to help with return to school may include:

- Starting school later, only going for half days, or going only to certain classes
- More time to finish assignments/tests
- Quiet room to finish assignments/tests
- Not going to noisy areas like the cafeteria, assembly halls, sporting events, music class, shop class, etc.

- Taking lots of breaks during class, homework, tests
- No more than one exam/day
- Shorter assignments
- Repetition/memory cues
- Use of a student helper/tutor
- Reassurance from teachers that the child will be supported while getting better

The child should not go back to sports until they are back to school/learning, without symptoms getting significantly worse and no longer needing any changes to their schedule.

© Concussion in Sport Group 2017

8

Sport concussion assessment tool for childrens ages 5 to 12 years

Br J Sports Med published online April 26, 2017

Updated information and services can be found at:
http://bjsm.bmj.com/content/early/2017/04/28/bjsports-2017-097492c
hildscat5.citation

These include:

Notes

BJSM Online First, published on April 26, 2017 as 10.1136/bjsports-2017-097508CRT5

To download a clean version of the SCAT tools please visit the journal online (http://dx.doi.org/10.1136/bjsports-2017-097508CRT5)

APPENDIX 2.3: THE CONCUSSION RECOGNITION TOOL 5

CONCUSSION RECOGNITION TOOL 5 ©

To help identify concussion in children, adolescents and adults

Supported by

FIFA® · [IIHF] · [IOC] · [World Rugby] · FEI

RECOGNISE & REMOVE

Head impacts can be associated with serious and potentially fatal brain injuries. The Concussion Recognition Tool 5 (CRT5) is to be used for the identification of suspected concussion. It is not designed to diagnose concussion.

STEP 1: RED FLAGS — CALL AN AMBULANCE

If there is concern after an injury including whether ANY of the following signs are observed or complaints are reported then the player should be safely and immediately removed from play/game/activity. If no licensed healthcare professional is available, call an ambulance for urgent medical assessment:

- Neck pain or tenderness
- Double vision
- Weakness or tingling/ burning in arms or legs
- Severe or increasing headache
- Seizure or convulsion
- Loss of consciousness
- Deteriorating conscious state
- Vomiting
- Increasingly restless, agitated or combative

Remember:

- In all cases, the basic principles of first aid (danger, response, airway, breathing, circulation) should be followed.
- Assessment for a spinal cord injury is critical.
- Do not attempt to move the player (other than required for airway support) unless trained to so do.
- Do not remove a helmet or any other equipment unless trained to do so safely.

If there are no Red Flags, identification of possible concussion should proceed to the following steps:

STEP 2: OBSERVABLE SIGNS

Visual clues that suggest possible concussion include:

- Lying motionless on the playing surface
- Slow to get up after a direct or indirect hit to the head
- Disorientation or confusion, or an inability to respond appropriately to questions
- Blank or vacant look
- Balance, gait difficulties, motor incoordination, stumbling, slow laboured movements
- Facial injury after head trauma

© Concussion In Sport Group 2017

STEP 3: SYMPTOMS

- Headache
- "Pressure in head"
- Balance problems
- Nausea or vomiting
- Drowsiness
- Dizziness
- Blurred vision
- Sensitivity to light
- Sensitivity to noise
- Fatigue or low energy
- "Don't feel right"
- More emotional
- More irritable
- Sadness
- Nervous or anxious
- Neck Pain
- Difficulty concentrating
- Difficulty remembering
- Feeling slowed down
- Feeling like "in a fog"

STEP 4: MEMORY ASSESSMENT

(IN ATHLETES OLDER THAN 12 YEARS)

Failure to answer any of these questions (modified appropriately for each sport) correctly may suggest a concussion:

- "What venue are we at today?"
- "Which half is it now?"
- "Who scored last in this game?"
- "What team did you play last week/game?"
- "Did your team win the last game?"

Athletes with suspected concussion should:

- Not be left alone initially (at least for the first 1–2 hours).
- Not drink alcohol.
- Not use recreational/ prescription drugs.
- Not be sent home by themselves. They need to be with a responsible adult.
- Not drive a motor vehicle until cleared to do so by a healthcare professional.

The CRT5 may be freely copied in its current form for distribution to individuals, teams, groups and organisations. Any revision and any reproduction in a digital form requires approval by the Concussion in Sport Group. It should not be altered in any way, rebranded or sold for commercial profit.

ANY ATHLETE WITH A SUSPECTED CONCUSSION SHOULD BE IMMEDIATELY REMOVED FROM PRACTICE OR PLAY AND SHOULD NOT RETURN TO ACTIVITY UNTIL ASSESSED MEDICALLY, EVEN IF THE SYMPTOMS RESOLVE

© Concussion in Sport Group 2017

© Concussion in Sport Group 2017

Davis GA, et al. Br J Sports Med 2017;0:1. doi:10.1136/bjsports-2017-097508CRT5

1

Concussion recognition tool 5©

Br J Sports Med published online April 26, 2017

Updated information and services can be found at:
**http://bjsm.bmj.com/content/early/2017/04/26/bjsports-2017-097508C
RT5.citation**

These include:

Email alerting service	Receive free email alerts when new articles cite this article. Sign up in the box at the top right corner of the online article.

Notes

To request permissions go to:
http://group.bmj.com/group/rights-licensing/permissions

To order reprints go to:
http://journals.bmj.com/cgi/reprintform

To subscribe to BMJ go to:
http://group.bmj.com/subscribe/

Further Reading

1) Putukian M, Schepart Z. Sideline assessment of concussion. In Hainline B, Stern RA (Eds.), *Sports Neurology*, San Diego: Elsevier BV, 2018, pp 75–80.

2) McCrory P, Meeuwisse W, Dvorak J, et al. Consensus statement on concussion in sport—the 5th international conference on concussion in sport held in Berlin, October 2016. *Br J Sports Med* 2017;51:838–847.

3) Echemendia RJ, Meeuwisse W, McCrory P, et al. The Sport Concussion Assessment Tool 5th Edition (SCAT5): background and rationale. *Br J Sports Med* 2017;51:848–850.

4) Davis GA, Purcell L, Schneider KJ, et al. The Child Sport Concussion Assessment Tool 5th Edition (Child SCAT5): background and rationale. *Br J Sports Med* 2017;51:859–861.

5) Zuckerman SL, Kerr ZY, Yengo-Kahn A, et al. Epidemiology of sports-related concussion in NCAA athletes from 2009–2010 to 2013–2014: incidence, recurrence, and mechanisms. *Am J Sports Med* 2015;43:2654–2662.

3 Acute Concussion and Cervical Spine Injury (John is not moving his legs after a tackle)

A 21-year-old male football player was lying motionless following a collision. The athlete had attempted to make a tackle, and he lowered his head to initiate contact. The opposing player also had his head lowered, and a helmet-to-helmet collision occurred. The athlete in question lay motionless, and upon evaluation, it was evident that he could not move his legs.

What do you do now?

CONCUSSION AND CERVICAL SPINE INJURY

Initial evaluation of an injured athlete should always include an assessment for the possibility of a more severe injury. This is especially true in concussion. If a direct or indirect impact to the head is severe enough to cause a concussion, it is also potentially severe enough to cause cervical spine injury. Although cervical spine injuries have diminished in football with the elimination of "spearing," such injuries persist in football and other high-risk sports, including cheerleading, gymnastics, equestrian, ice hockey, pole vaulting, and more.

Neurologic compromise from cervical spine injury can progress rapidly, so proper initial management is critical. All athletes involved in a collision injury should be assessed for the possibility of cervical spinal cord injury. This initial assessment is pivotal, as it leads to a decision to proceed (or not) with cervical spine stabilization. "Red flags" for cervical spinal cord injury include altered consciousness, point tenderness along the cervical spine, obvious cervical spine bony deformity, and extremity motor and/or sensory deficits (Box 3.1). Unilateral arm weakness more commonly develops as a result of a burner or stinger, which is seen in awake athletes who are otherwise not compromised but had an acute traction injury to the brachial plexus. This injury is more common after tackling or blocking in football and is generally self-limiting.

If cervical spine injury is suspected, the emergency action plan for spinal stabilization should be enacted. Ideally, emergency action plans are rehearsed regularly, and a mini-rehearsal occurs before the sporting event (Box 3.2). Although spine stabilization techniques are beyond the scope of this book, basic manual in-line stabilization can be performed by any provider. One method is to place the fingertips beneath the mastoid processes and wrap both hands around the occiput. The other is to grasp the trapezii

---

BOX 3.1. **"Red Flags" for Proceeding to Cervical Spine Stabilization**

Altered consciousness
Complaints of cervical spine pain or focal spine tenderness
Cervical spinal deformity
Extremity motor and/or sensory deficits

BOX 3.2. The Emergency Action Plan

Annual rehearsal
Mini-rehearsal that is venue-specific
Identification of nearest trauma center/emergency medical services
Team leader and team members
Proper equipment
    Backboard
    Cervical collar
    Scissors
    Helmet/shoulder pad/facemask removal tools, where appropriate
    Airway management devices
    Automatic external defibrillator

---

with the hands and secure the head between the forearms. Airway access always takes precedence, as individuals can deteriorate rapidly following respiratory arrest. If a team is on site to perform primary spinal stabilization and backboard placement, then they should proceed. Otherwise, emergency medical services should be activated, while continuing the best attempt to maintain manual in-line spinal stabilization.

TAKE-HOME POINTS

- Always have a low threshold for suspecting cervical spine injury in concussed athletes.
- Emergency action plans should be rehearsed.
- If cervical spine injury is suspected, manual in-line stabilization should proceed.
- Airway access is a primary concern in injuries serious enough to cause cervical spine injury.

Further Reading

1) Blatz D, Ross B, Dadabo J. Cervical spine trauma evaluation. In Hainline B, Stern RA (Eds.), *Sports Neurology*, San Diego: Elsevier BV, 2018, pp 345–351.

2) Boissy P, Shrier I, Briere S, et al. Effectiveness of cervical spine stabilization techniques. *Clin J Sport Med* 2011;21:80–88.

3) Ahn H, Singh J, Nathens A, et al. Pre-hospital care management of a potential spinal cord injured patients: a systematic review of the literature and evidence-based guidelines. *J Neurotrauma* 2011;28:1341–1361.

4 Acute Concussion versus Catastrophic Brain Injury (Elizabeth struck her head and is increasingly sleepy)

An 18-year-old cheerleader was practicing for an upcoming game. She was rehearsing a pyramid formation, lost her balance, and struck her head on the asphalt pavement. There was no mat in place. She immediately complained of headache, but otherwise was initially alert. About one hour later, she became drowsy, and within the next 30 minutes fell into a coma. She was airlifted to a Level I trauma center.

What do you do now?

CATASTROPHIC BRAIN INJURY

As stated elsewhere in this book, if an injury is severe enough to cause a concussion, it is potentially severe enough to cause a more serious injury to the brain or cervical spine. Concussion is a type of mild traumatic brain injury, and is on a continuum that includes moderate and severe traumatic brain injuries. Such injuries are determined in part by the force of impact, and the nature and location of the impact. Simplistically, the force of impact is measured as either a linear or rotational acceleration, but most impacts are a combination of both.

In addition to the initial severity of the impact force, the location of the injury must be considered. For example, an epidural hematoma may develop following a fracture to the temporal bone, with subsequent shearing of the middle meningeal artery, resulting in a hematoma between the skull and dura mater. This rapidly evolving injury is not necessarily from a more severe impact, but rather from a strategically located fracture of the temporal bone.

Individuals who suffer a head injury require serial monitoring. Not only may concussion symptomatology evolve over time, but intra- or extracranial brain hemorrhage may evolve over minutes to hours. Because such hemorrhages are an expanding mass in an enclosed space (the skull), there is increasing pressure on the brain, which can lead to devastating consequences. An emergency action plan must be activated in any of these scenarios following concussion:

- Glasgow Coma Scale < 13
- Prolonged loss of consciousness
- Focal neurological deficit consistent with intracranial trauma
- Repeated vomiting
- Persistently diminished or worsening mental status/level of consciousness
- Persistently diminished or worsening neurologic symptoms and signs.

The National Center for Catastrophic Sport Injury Research at the University of North Carolina at Chapel Hill has monitored catastrophic injury in sports since 1982. They classify such injuries as *traumatic* (direct) or *nontraumatic* (indirect or exertional) injuries. Catastrophic brain injuries result from brain trauma. Football has the highest number of traumatic brain injuries of any sport, but other high-risk sports include gymnastics, skiing, and ice hockey. Prompt recognition is pivotal to acute management, but the primary focus should be on preventing such injuries (Box 4.1).

Catastrophic brain injuries from sport are most commonly described as epidural or subdural hematoma, or subarachnoid or intracranial hemorrhage. Second impact syndrome will be discussed in the next chapter. On-site management centers on having a low threshold for making a diagnosis and activating an emergency action plan. As with all emergencies, breathing, airway, and circulation must be monitored and maintained. On-site management otherwise consists of maintaining calm while activating the emergency action plan with rapid transport to a trauma center.

TAKE-HOME POINTS

· Moderate and severe catastrophic brain injuries exist on a continuum with concussion and mild traumatic brain injury.

· Head injury severe enough to cause a concussion may be severe enough to cause moderate or severe brain injury.

· An emergency action plan must be activated when there is any suspicion of a catastrophic brain injury.

Further Reading

1) Wolff CS, Cantu RC, Kucera KL. Catastrophic neurologic injuries in sport. In Hainline B, Stern RA (Eds.), *Sports Neurology*, San Diego: Elsevier BV, 2018, pp 25–37.

2) National Collegiate Athletic Association (2017). NCAA catastrophic sport injury reporting FAQS, Indianapolis, IN. http://www.ncaa.org/sport-science-institue/ ncaa-catastrophic-sport-injury-reporting-faqs. Accessed March 28, 2019.

3) Kucera KL, Yau RK, Register-Mihalik J, et al. Traumatic brain and spinal cord fatalities among high school and college football players—United States, 2005–2014. *MMWR Morb Mortal Wkl Rep* 2017;65a;1465–1469.

5 Acute Concussion versus Second Impact Syndrome (Fred is posturing on the ice after colliding with another player)

A 17-year-old male hockey player fell onto the ice after colliding with another player. The collision did not appear to be high impact, i.e., there was not a major observed collision force to the head, nor was there a major collision force when he fell to the ice. He lay motionless and unresponsive, and within minutes developed decorticate and then decerebrate posturing. The player was immediately evaluated and transferred appropriately to a trauma center.

What do you do now?

SECOND IMPACT SYNDROME

Second impact syndrome is an exceedingly rare condition that lacks a clear definition. The term "second impact" was first utilized in the context of contact sports in a 1984 case report of a football player who died four days after a head injury. Subsequently, Cantu and others have popularized the term "second impact syndrome."

Second impact syndrome is one of the most poorly understood manifestations of head injury, yet it has generated considerable media attention and has become the basis of many concussion laws. Indeed, in the United States all 50 states now have a law in place which prevents an athlete from returning to the field of play on the same day of the diagnosed concussion. These laws stem from a movement in Washington following a devastating neurologic injury to a young football player, Zachery Lystedt. In 2006, Zach hit his head while making a tackle, and minutes later returned to the game. After the game, he collapsed and was air transported to Seattle's Harborview Medical Center, and was treated for a brain herniation secondary to brain hemorrhage. He suffered permanent neurologic injury, and his case was a springboard for media and policy attention to the potentially devastating effects of head injury in contact/collision sports.

Zachery Lystedt suffered from brain hemorrhage and brain swelling after his injury. Second impact syndrome describes a head injury that occurs in the setting of a prior head injury in which symptoms had not fully cleared. It is assumed that the second impact in an unrecovered brain leads to a severe malfunction of cerebral autoregulation, with subsequent massive brain swelling and brain herniation. There are only 17 documented cases of second impact syndrome in the literature, and only 5 involved a well-documented repeat head injury. In tracing cases that went to autopsy, most had other structural brain injuries, such as intracranial bleeding. Thus, whether second impact syndrome is a unique clinical and pathologic entity remains uncertain.

Some have argued that second impact syndrome is likely to be linked to a genetic predisposition to cerebral dysautoregulation. Regardless, some athletes can develop catastrophic consequences from head injury, and the underlying mechanism is not clear. We need further research regarding genetics, repetitive head impact exposure versus clinical concussion, and the scientific meaning of neurobiological recovery following head injury.

As noted previously, there is ample reason to mitigate exposure to head injury, and to always have in place a well-rehearsed emergency action plan in contact/collision sport venues. If second impact syndrome is suspected, there should be immediate activation of an emergency action plan with transport to a Level I trauma center, similar to the management of catastrophic brain injuries noted in Chapter 4.

TAKE-HOME POINTS

· Second impact syndrome is a head injury that occurs when recovery from a prior head injury is incomplete.
· Second impact syndrome refers to uncontrolled cerebral edema that leads to brain herniation.
· Second impact syndrome is exceedingly rare, and the cause is uncertain.

Further Reading

1) Saunders RI, Harbaugh RE. The second impact in catastrophic contact-sports head trauma. *JAMA* 1984;252:538–539.

2) Cantu RC. Second impact syndrome: immediate management. *Phys Sportsmed* 1992;20:55–66.

3) Wolff CS, Cantu RC, Kucera KL. Catastrophic neurologic injuries in sport. In Hainline B, Stern RA (Eds.), *Sports Neurology*, San Diego: Elsevier BV, 2018, pp 25–37.

4) Stovitz S, Weseman J, Hooks MC, et al. What definition is used to describe second impact syndrome in sports? A systematic and critical review. *Curr Sports Med Rep* 2017;16:50–55.

5) McCrory P, Gavin D, Makdissi M. Second impact syndrome or cerebral swelling after sporting head injury. *Curr Sports Med Rep* 2012;11:21–23.

6 Concussion One Hour Later (Betty is becoming more confused while sitting on the sideline)

A 23-year-old lacrosse player lost her balance, fell, and struck her head on the ground. She arose slowly, and seemed to be stumbling while returning to the sideline. The athletic trainer immediately suspected a sport-related concussion and insisted that Betty be evaluated further. As this was a championship game, and Betty was a star player, she argued repeatedly that she was fine and would not undergo an evaluation. The athletic trainer did not allow her to return to play without first administering a SCAT5 questionnaire. His suspicions of concussion were confirmed, and he instructed Betty to remain on the sideline. One hour later, she became more confused. She had no complaints of headache, and she had no segmental or balance symptoms or signs.

What do you do now?

CONCUSSION ONE HOUR LATER

This case illustrates that concussion is not a singular event, but rather a process. It is worth examining two recently proposed definitions of concussion.

The American Medical Society for Sports Medicine position statement on concussion defines concussion as a traumatically induced transient disturbance of brain function that involves a complex pathophysiological process. Note that *process* is a key part of this definition.

The Fifth International Conference on Concussion in Sport provides a more detailed definition of concussion, which is noted in Box 6.1. Importantly, this definition states the following: sport-related concussion typically results in the rapid onset of short-lived impairment of neurologic function that resolves spontaneously. However, in some cases, signs and symptoms evolve over a number of minutes to hours. Note that *evolve* is a key part of this definition.

Although there is emerging information that acute concussion can lead to structural changes in the brain—including loss of white matter integrity, cerebral microhemorrhage, and axonal disruption—most scientists and clinicians continue to describe concussion as a functional disturbance rather than a structural injury per se. Yet it is the functional nature of concussion that can lead to an evolution of symptoms. If a mechanical force reaches a critical threshold (which remains undefined), the result is a temporary disruption of cellular membranes, with subsequent indiscriminate release of neurotransmitters. Potassium and glutamate increase in the extracellular space, and calcium accumulates in the intracellular space. The ATPase pump is activated to re-establish ionic equilibrium, which requires an increase in cerebral glucose metabolism. This response is then coupled with a biphasic metabolic response, which leads to a decrease in glucose metabolism. This neural-metabolic cascade may evolve over minutes to hours, and thus the clinical manifestation of concussion may evolve over minutes to hours.

It is further speculated that the "hyperfocus" of athletes playing in a championship event may mask some early concussion symptoms. Thus, it is highly recommended that athletes with suspected sport-related concussion be evaluated away from the field of play, in a quiet space. The SCAT5 takes approximately 10 minutes to administer, and this extra time allows for a better assessment of possible concussion.

BOX 6.1. **Definition of Concussion by the 2017 Concussion in Sport Group Consensus Statement**

Sport-related concussion (SRC) is a traumatic brain injury induced by biomechanical forces. Common features that may be utilized in clinically defining the nature of a concussive head injury include the following:

· SRC may be caused either by a direct blow to the head, face, or neck, or elsewhere on the body with an impulsive force transmitted to the head.
· SRC typically results in the rapid onset of short-lived impairment of neurological function that resolves spontaneously. However, in some cases, signs and symptoms evolve over a number of minutes to hours.
· SRC may result in neuropathological changes, but the acute clinical signs and symptoms largely reflect a functional disturbance rather than a structural injury and, as such, no abnormality is seen on standard structural neuroimaging studies.
· SRC results in a range of clinical signs and symptoms that may or may not involve loss of consciousness. Resolution of the clinical and cognitive features typically follows a sequential course. However, in some cases symptoms may be prolonged.

The clinical signs and symptoms cannot be explained by drug, alcohol, or medication use, other injuries (cervical injuries, peripheral vestibular dysfunction, etc.) or other comorbidities (e.g., psychological factors or coexisting medical conditions).

There should always be a low threshold for suspecting sport-related concussion, and if concussion is suspected, not only must the athlete not return to competition or play that same day; he or she also must be observed over time. It should be expected that concussion symptoms may evolve over minutes to hours. This knowledge provides reassurance that an athlete is not developing a yet more serious traumatic brain injury, but does not obviate the need for assessing for this possibility.

An important part of concussion management is to manage expectations. Clinicians, coaches, stakeholders, and athletes should all be aware of the definition of concussion, and should understand that clinicians must always have a low threshold for making this diagnosis. They must further understand that because concussion is a process, symptoms may evolve over minutes to hours.

TAKE-HOME POINTS

- Concussion is best understood as a neurologic process, not a singular event.
- Concussion is primarily the result of a neural-metabolic cascade that evolves over time.
- Concussion symptoms may worsen over minutes to hours, and so athletes with suspected concussion should be monitored serially.
- There must always be a low threshold for diagnosing sport-related concussion.
- A sideline neurologic exam is best performed in a quiet environment.
- Any athlete with a suspected concussion must not be allowed to return to play or competition that same day.

Further Reading

1) Harmon KG, Clugston JR, Dec K, et al. American Medical Society for Sports Medicine position statement on concussion in sport. *Br J Sports Med* 2019;53:213–225.

2) McCrory P, Meeuwisse W, Dvorak J, et al. Consensus statement on concussion in sport—the 5th international conference on concussion in sport held in Berlin, October 2016. *Br J Sports Med* 2017;51:838–847.

3) Giza C, Greco T, Prins ML. Concussion: pathophysiology and clinical translation. In Hainline B, Stern RA (Eds.), *Sports Neurology*, San Diego: Elsevier BV, 2018, pp 51–61.

7 Concussion Two Weeks Later (Something is not right)

A 35-year-old man suffered a concussion while training in mixed martial arts. He received a kick to the head that resulted in a witnessed rapid rotation of his head from left to right. He did not fall, but stumbled over the next several minutes, complaining of considerable dizziness. He was confused, had very poor memory regarding his current circumstances (including where he was, and why he was in a gym without shoes). He was taken to the Emergency Department, where he was evaluated, diagnosed with a concussion, and sent home with nonspecific post-concussion instructions. When he was re-evaluated by his primary care physician two weeks later, he had considerable complaints of dizziness without vertigo, poor short-term memory, and difficulty falling asleep.

What do you do now?

CONCUSSION TWO WEEKS LATER

Concussion is considered a condition in which complete recovery can be expected in over 80% of athletes over 7–10 days. This trajectory is based on a study of male collegiate football players in the United States, evaluated in a well-confined environment. Yet up to 20% of athletes did not recover during this period, and the reasons are not well defined. Predictors of more prolonged recovery are only now beginning to emerge, and include the following:

- Loss of consciousness
- Post-traumatic amnesia
- Greater number of acute symptoms
- Immediate complaints of dizziness.

This group with more prolonged recovery requires special attention and is the focus of the next two chapters of this book. Although prolonged recovery is becoming more predictable based on symptoms, there are no objective biomarker predictors of prolonged recovery. To date, there is a paucity of evidence regarding the neurobiology of concussion, including acute and subacute injury, and possible prolonged sequelae of concussion. Although the emergence of subjective symptoms as a predictor of prolonged recovery is important in managing expectations, it remains insufficient with regard to understanding brain mechanisms of recovery.

Further complicating prediction of prolonged recovery is the presence of other risk factors, such as genetics, age, numbers of prior concussions and prior exposures to repetitive head impacts, and comorbid neuropsychiatric conditions. Additionally, data have emerged recently regarding the impact of acute intervention on prolonged recovery.

It is important to discuss the fear that overwhelms many individuals who present with prolonged post-concussion recovery. It is commonplace for sports medicine clinicians, including sports neurologists, to be deluged with questions regarding the possibility of developing chronic traumatic encephalopathy or another neurodegenerative condition as a result of concussion. This fear, and associated anxiety, can further intermingle with prolonged recovery because anxiety can cause persistent symptoms following concussion, as discussed later in this book.

The discerning clinician who is evaluating a patient with prolonged recovery from concussion must consider the following:

- An understanding of the initial concussive injury, with attention to immediate symptoms and signs
- A checklist for any "red flags" (see Box 2.1, Chapter 2)
- A review of the individual's understanding of concussion, with special attention to unfounded fears regarding this condition
- A review of the level of activity that the individual has engaged in since the concussive injury
- A focused neuropsychiatric exam to assess the possibility of emerging persistent post-concussion symptoms, or emerging mental health symptoms and disorders
- Management recommendations that address these factors.

If the clinical encounter two weeks following concussion reveals prolonged recovery, and the overall profile is consistent simply with a heavy symptom burden at the time of injury, then the patient can be reassured, and a rational return to activity can be prescribed. If the encounter reveals worrisome neurologic signs, then neuroimaging and other tests, as indicated, should be recommended. If the return to activity protocol has been wholly unsatisfactory, then this should be addressed. Similarly, if comorbid neurologic conditions have not been managed or are emerging, these too should be addressed. Finally, any emerging mental health symptoms or disorders also should be addressed. All of these issues are discussed in the chapters that follow.

TAKE-HOME POINTS

- Although most individuals with concussion recover in 7–10 days, this information is based on a study of male US collegiate football athletes.
- Loss of consciousness, post-traumatic amnesia, increased symptoms, and acute dizziness predict prolonged recovery.
- There are no objective neurobiologic predictors of prolonged recovery.
- The discerning clinician must differentiate expected prolonged recovery from worrisome traumatic brain injury or unaddressed neuropsychiatric conditions.

Further Reading

1) McCrea M, Guskiewicz KM, Marshall S, et al. Acute effects and recovery time following concussion in collegiate football players. The NCAA Concussion Study. *JAMA* 2003;290:2556–2563.

2) McCrea M, Guskiewicz K, Randolph C, et al. Incidence, clinical course, and predictors of prolonged recovery time following sport-related concussion in high school and college athletes. *J Int Neuropsych Soc* 2013;19:22–33.

3) Charek DB, Collins M, Kontos A. Office-based concussion evaluation, diagnosis, and management: adult. In Hainline B, Stern RA (Eds.), *Sports Neurology*, San Diego: Elsevier BV, 2018, pp 91–105.

4) Paquin H, Taylor A, Meehan WP. Office-based concussion evaluation, diagnosis, and management: pediatric. In Hainline B, Stern RA (Eds). *Sports Neurology,* San Diego: Elsevier BV, 2018, pp 107–117.

8 Return to Learn Following Concussion (I can't concentrate in school)

A 14-year-old girl suffered a concussion after slipping at a bowling alley. She had just released the bowling ball, lost her balance, and fell, striking the side of her head. She developed an immediate headache and complained of dizziness. She was evaluated the next day by her primary care physician, who diagnosed an "uncomplicated concussion." He recommended that she return to her activities, including school, as tolerated. No specific accommodations or stepwise increases in activity were provided. She was re-evaluated one week later because she could not concentrate while in school.

What do you do now?

RETURN TO LEARN FOLLOWING CONCUSSION

We must always remember that children, adolescents, and emerging adults who suffer from concussion are also students. Whereas much of the literature and media attention have focused on when athletes should return to play, there has been much less literature regarding returning to school following a concussion. In 2013, the American Academy of Pediatrics was the first medical organization to address this matter, and their recommendations became a springboard for subsequent return-to-learn strategies. In 2014, the NCAA published a "checklist" based on an interassociation best practices document that included return-to-learn recommendations. The Centers for Disease Control and Prevention published return-to-learn recommendations for school administrators.

Concussion is not a homogeneous entity, and individuals may present with various symptoms, including headache, dizziness, difficulty concentrating, difficulty reading, fatigue, and mood disorders. All these symptoms can impair a student's performance in the classroom. An individualized plan should be developed for each patient to return to school. Management of this stage has evolved from recommendations of cognitive rest until asymptomatic to multidisciplinary plans that include an understanding of the patient's underlying symptomatology. Whereas most individuals can become fully reintegrated into an academic setting with nonspecific recommendations, it is preferable to consider the following key points when making return-to-learn recommendations:

1) An individualized return-to-learn plan should be developed for all students who have suffered a concussion. Such a plan manages expectations for students, parents, and teachers. This plan should be transparent, to allow any deviation from the plan to be addressed and corrected as needed. Appendix 8.1 is an example of a template that can be used for students who are returning to school following concussion.

2) Academic accommodations become necessary when more informal academic adjustments are not adequate. These adjustments can be made through either a 504 plan or an individualized education plan (IEP). Both of these plans are protected through the American with Disabilities Education Act.

Appendix 8.2 is a formal checklist that is the basis for all concussion safety protocols of NCAA member schools. Importantly, the return-to-learn component of the checklist recommends a multidisciplinary approach, and a re-evaluation of all students who remain symptomatic for two weeks following concussion. The recommendation for such a formal re-evaluation is meant to mitigate prolonged recovery secondary to comorbid or emerging neuropsychiatric conditions.

TAKE-HOME POINTS

- Students who suffer with concussion may develop several symptoms that interfere with returning to school.
- Clinicians should address the return-to-learn plan in a transparent manner that manages expectations for students, parents, and teachers.
- Most individuals can successfully navigate returning to school through an informal, individualized management plan.
- Students having difficulty returning to school should be re-evaluated at two weeks following concussion to assess for the possibility of emerging comorbid neuropsychiatric conditions.
- More formal management plans should be developed for students with prolonged return-to-learn difficulties.

APPENDIX 8.1: TEMPLATE FOR SCHOOL RECOMMENDATIONS FOLLOWING CONCUSSION

SCHOOL RECOMMENDATIONS FOLLOWING CONCUSSION

Patient Name: _____   Date of Birth: _____
Date of Evaluation: _____   Referred by: _____
Duration of Recommendations: 1 week   2 weeks   4 weeks   Until further notice

The patient will be reassessed for revision of these recommendations in _____ weeks.

This patient has been diagnosed with a concussion (a brain injury) and is currently under our care. Please excuse the patient from school today due to the medical appointment. Flexibility and additional supports are needed during recovery. The following are suggestions for academic adjustments to be individualized for the student as deemed appropriate in the school setting. Feel free to apply/remove adjustments as needed as the student's symptoms improve/worsen.

Attendance
_____   No school for ____ school day(s)
_____   Attendance at school ____ days per week
_____   Full school days as tolerated by the student as
_____   Partial days as tolerated by the student personnel

Breaks
_____   Allow the student to go to the nurse's office if symptoms increase
_____   Allow other breaks during the school day

deemed necessary and appropriate by school

Visual Stimulus
_____   Change classroom seating as necessary
_____   Pre-printed notes for class material or note taker
_____   Avoid extremes of light/dark in classrooms
_____   Reduce brightness on monitors/screens

Audible Stimulus
_____   Lunch in a quiet place with a friend
_____   Avoid music or shop classes
_____   Allow to wear earplugs as needed

Workload/Multi-Tasking
_____   Reduce overall amount of make-up work, class work and homework
_____   Prorate workload when possible
_____   Reduce amount of homework given each night
_____   Excuse from makeup work if possible

Testing
_____   Additional time to complete tests
_____   No more than one test a day
_____   No standardized testing until _____
_____   Allow for scribe, oral response, and oral delivery of questions, if available

Physical Exertion
_____   No physical exertion/athletics/gym/recess
_____   Walking in gym class only
_____   Begin return to play protocol as outlined by return to activity form

Additional Recommendations
_____
_____
_____
_____

Current Symptoms List (the student is noting these today)
_____ Headache	_____ Visual problems	_____ Sensitivity to noise	_____ Memory issues
_____ Nausea	_____ Balance problems	_____ Feeling foggy	_____ Fatigue
_____ Dizziness	_____ Sensitivity to light	_____ Difficulty concentrating	_____ Irritability

Student is reporting most difficulty with/in
_____ All subjects	_____ Reading/Language arts	_____ Foreign Language	_____ Math
_____ Science	_____ Music	_____ History	_____ Using Computers
_____ Focusing	_____ Listening	Other: _____	

Reprinted with permission, Sports Neurology, 2018.

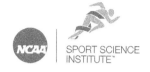

CONCUSSION SAFETY
PROTOCOL CHECKLIST

Below is a checklist that will help the athletics health care administrator ensure that the member school's concussion safety protocol is compliant with the Concussion Safety Protocol Legislation and is consistent with Interassociation Consensus: Diagnosis and Management of Sport-Related Concussion Best Practices.

Please do not hesitate to reach out to Brian Hainline (NCAA chief medical officer and administrative chair of the committee) at ssi@ncaa.org if you have any questions or concerns. The committee's primary purpose is to serve as an advocate for promoting and developing concussion safety management plans for each member school.

Last revised: March 2017

1

PRESEASON EDUCATION:

Education management plan that specifies:

☐ Institution has provided NCAA concussion fact sheets (NCAA will make the material available) or other applicable material annually to the following parties:

  ☐ Student-athletes.

  ☐ Coaches.

  ☐ Team physicians.

  ☐ Athletic trainers.

  ☐ Directors of athletics.

☐ Each party provides a signed acknowledgment of having read and understood the concussion material.

2

PRE-PARTICIPATION ASSESSMENT:

Pre-participation management plan that specifies:

❑ Documentation that each varsity student-athlete has received at least one pre-participation baseline concussion assessment that addresses:

  ❑ Brain injury and concussion history.

  ❑ Symptom evaluation.

  ❑ Cognitive assessment.

  ❑ Balance evaluation.

  ❑ Team physician determines pre-participation clearance and/or the need for additional consultation or testing.*

Consider a new baseline concussion assessment six months or beyond for any varsity student-athlete with a documented concussion, especially those with complicated or multiple concussion history.

RECOGNITION AND DIAGNOSIS OF CONCUSSION:

Recognition and diagnosis of concussion management plan that specifies:

☐ Medical personnel with training in the diagnosis, treatment and initial management of acute concussion must be "present" at all NCAA varsity competitions in the following contact/collision sports: basketball; equestrian; field hockey; football; ice hockey; lacrosse; pole vault; rugby; skiing; soccer; wrestling. To be present means to be on site at the campus or arena of the competition. Medical personnel may be from either team, or may be independently contracted for the event.

☐ Medical personnel with training in the diagnosis, treatment and initial management of acute concussion must be "available" at all NCAA varsity practices in the following contact/collision sports: basketball; equestrian; field hockey; football; ice hockey; lacrosse; pole vault; rugby; skiing; soccer; wrestling. To be available means that, at a minimum, medical personnel can be contacted at any time during the practice via telephone, messaging, email, beeper or other immediate communication means. Further, the case can be discussed through such communication, and immediate arrangements can be made for the athlete to be evaluated.

☐ Any student-athlete with signs/symptoms/behaviors consistent with concussion:

   ☐ Must be removed from practice or competition.

   ☐ Must be evaluated by an athletic trainer or team physician with concussion experience.

   ☐ Must be removed from practice/play for that calendar day if concussion is confirmed.

4

NCAA Sport Science Institute
Concussion Safety Protocol Checklist

Initial suspected concussion evaluation management plan that specifies:

- ❏ Symptom assessment.

- ❏ Physical and neurological exam.

- ❏ Cognitive assessment.

- ❏ Balance exam.

- ❏ Clinical assessment for cervical spine trauma, skull fracture and intracranial bleed.

5

POST-CONCUSSION MANAGEMENT:

Post-concussion management plan that specifies:

☐ Emergency action plan, including transportation for further medical care, for any of the following:

    ☐ Glasgow Coma Scale < 13.

    ☐ Prolonged loss of consciousness.

    ☐ Focal neurological deficit suggesting intracranial trauma.

    ☐ Repetitive emesis.

    ☐ Persistently diminished/worsening mental status or other neurological signs/symptoms.

    ☐ Spine injury.

☐ Mechanism for serial evaluation and monitoring after injury.

☐ Documentation of oral and/or written care to both student-athlete and another responsible adult.*

May be parent or roommate.

☐ Evaluation by a physician for student-athlete with prolonged recovery in order to consider additional diagnosis* and best management options.

Additional diagnoses include, but are not limited to:

    ✻ *Post-concussion syndrome.*
    ✻ *Sleep dysfunction.*
    ✻ *Migraine or other headache disorders.*
    ✻ *Mood disorders such as anxiety and depression.*
    ✻ *Ocular or vestibular dysfunction.*

6

RETURN-TO-PLAY:

Return-to-play management plan that specifies:

☐ Final determination of return-to-play is from the team physician or medically qualified physician designee.

☐ Each student-athlete with a concussion must undergo a supervised stepwise progression management plan by a health care provider with expertise in concussion that specifies:

  ☐ Student-athlete has limited physical and cognitive activity until he/she has returned to baseline, then progresses with each step below without worsening or new symptoms:

    ☐ Light aerobic exercise without resistance training.

    ☐ Sport-specific exercise and activity without head impact.

    ☐ Non-contact practice with progressive resistance training.

    ☐ Unrestricted training.

    ☐ Return to competition.

7

RETURN-TO-LEARN:

<u>Return-to-learn</u> management plan that specifies:

☐ Identification of a point person within the athletics department who will navigate return-to-learn with the student-athlete.

☐ Identification of a multidisciplinary team* that will navigate more complex cases of prolonged return-to-learn:

Multidisciplinary team may include, but not be limited to:

> ❋ *Team physician.*
> ❋ *Athletic trainer.*
> ❋ *Psychologist/counselor.*
> ❋ *Neuropsychologist consultant.*
> ❋ *Faculty athletics representative.*
> ❋ *Academic counselor.*
> ❋ *Course instructor(s).*
> ❋ *College administrators.*
> ❋ *Office of disability services representatives.*
> ❋ *Coaches.*

☐ Compliance with ADAAA.

☐ No classroom activity on same day as the concussion.

☐ Individualized initial plan that includes:

  ☐ Remaining at home/dorm if the student-athlete cannot tolerate light cognitive activity.

  ☐ Gradual return to classroom/studying as tolerated.

☐ Re-evaluation by the team physician if concussion symptoms worsen with academic challenges.

8

NCAA Sport Science Institute
Concussion Safety Protocol Checklist

☐ Modification of schedule/academic accommodations for up to two weeks, as indicated, with help from the identified point person.

☐ Re-evaluation by the team physician and members of the multidisciplinary team, as appropriate, for a student-athlete with symptoms lasting longer than two weeks.

☐ Engaging campus resources for cases that cannot be managed through schedule modification/academic accommodations.

☐ Such campus resources must be consistent with ADAAA, and include at least one of the following:

* *Learning specialists.*
* *Office of disability services.*
* *ADAAA office.*

REDUCING EXPOSURE TO HEAD TRAUMA:

☐ <u>Reducing head trauma exposure</u> management plan.*

While the committee acknowledges that 'reducing' may be difficult to quantify, it is important to emphasize ways to minimize head trauma exposure. Examples of minimizing head trauma exposure include, but are not limited to:

* *Adherence to Interassociation Consensus: Year-Round Football Practice Contact Recommendations.*
* *Adherence to Interassociation Consensus: Independent Medical Care for College Student-Athletes Best Practices.*
* *Reducing gratuitous contact during practice.*
* *Taking a "safety-first" approach to sport.*
* *Taking the head out of contact.*
* *Coaching and student-athlete education regarding safe play and proper technique.*

9

ADMINISTRATIVE:

☐ Institutional plan submitted* to the Concussion Safety Protocol Committee by May 1.

Plans must be submitted via Program Hub.

☐ Written certificate of compliance signed by the athletics health care administrator that accompanies the submitted plan.

NCAA Sport Science Institute
Concussion Safety Protocol Checklist

Further Reading

1) Halstead ME. Return to learn. In Hainline B, Stern RA (Eds.), *Sports Neurology*, San Diego: Elsevier BV, 2018, pp 199–204.

2) Interassociation consensus: diagnosis and management of sport related concussion best practices. http://www.ncaa.org/sites/default/files/SSI_ConcussionBestPractices_20170616.pdf. Accessed March 29, 2019.

3) NCAA Concussion Safety Protocol Checklist. http://www.ncaa.org/sites/default/files/SSI_ConcussionProtocolCheckList_20180213.pdf. Accessed March 29, 2019.

4) Centers for Disease Control and Prevention. Returning to school after a concussion: a fact sheet for school professionals. https://www.cdc.gov/headsup/pdfs/schools/tbi_returning_to_school-a.pdf. Accessed September 14, 2019.

9   Return to Play Following Concussion (Each time I push myself I feel worse)

A 21-year-old male basketball player suffered a concussion while attempting a rebound. He received a sharp blow to the head from his opponent's elbow, lost his balance and fell, and his head struck the floor. He immediately felt dazed, disoriented, and dizzy, and walked aimlessly until guided by his teammates to the bench. He was removed from the game and evaluated in the locker room, and did not return to play that day. He was instructed to undergo a graduated return-to-play protocol after initial cognitive and physical rest. However, he chose instead to stay in his room for over one week because he felt so unwell. He did no physical activity during that time, and did not return to the classroom. When he attempted the return-to-play protocol, he developed increasing symptoms of feeling disoriented and dizzy.

What do you do now?

RETURN TO PLAY

Return-to-play protocols have been established since 1986. Between 1986 and 1997, three protocols from prominent organizations stressed a gradual return to play following concussion injury. Notably, all protocols allowed an athlete to return to play on the same day if initial concussion symptoms resolved within 15–20 minutes. More prolonged absence from competition or training was recommended for concussion that resulted in more prolonged symptoms, or that resulted in loss of consciousness. The Concussion in Sport Group, which has issued international guidelines every four years since 2001, has developed a "gold standard" protocol for graduated return to play following concussion. However, the medical literature has provided conflicting recommendations through 2012, with peer-reviewed articles in some prominent journals recommending same-day return to play through the first decade of the twenty-first century. It was not until 2012 that the Concussion in Sport Group made an unqualified recommendation for no return to play on the same day as a concussion.

The cornerstone of initial management following concussion has been physical and cognitive rest. This is based on data from animal models showing that cerebral blood flow is reduced following concussion, and brain-derived neurotrophic factors worsen with forced exercise within one to two days of a concussion. Although physical and cognitive rest have become well accepted as the mainstream of initial concussion management during the past several years, there is also emerging clinical evidence that many patients were subjected to prolonged cognitive and physical rest, so-called cocoon therapy. Emerging information has demonstrated that cocoon therapy harms concussion recovery. Indeed, after 48 hours exercise promotes release of brain-derived neurotrophic factors, and is an effective treatment for many common mental health symptoms following concussion, including disordered sleep, depression, anxiety, and nonspecific fatigue. Such emerging information has led to a fundamental shift in return-to-play protocols, such that early exercise following concussion is now recommended.

Another shift developed because many clinicians recommended that a return-to-play protocol could not begin until the patient was asymptomatic. However, athletes often report baseline symptoms like those frequently described following concussion, such as a history of headache, sleep disorder, or mood disorder. Thus, it is now recommended that return-to-play protocols begin when prominent post-concussion symptoms are resolving, and individuals are returning to their baseline condition.

In the most recent position statement of the American Medical Society for Sports Medicine, and in the most recent consensus statement from the Concussion in Sport Group, aerobic exercise was recommended as early as 24–48 hours following concussion. These recommendations are based on emerging information that subsymptom threshold exercise improves recovery in acute concussion and that such intervention is safe.

Box 9.1 provides a summary of commonly accepted return-to-play protocols. With each stage, exercise and sport-specific activities are introduced, with at least a 24-hour window before beginning the next stage.

Ultimately, return to play is a balance between ensuring player safety and not augmenting persistent concussion symptoms because of inactivity. Premature return to play may increase the risk of a subsequent concussion within 10 days of the initial injury. This information must be balanced with equally compelling emerging data that inadequate concussion management

---

BOX 9.1. **Standard Template for Return to Play**

Stage 1. Symptom-limited activity, with gradual introduction of daily activities.

Stage 2. Light aerobic exercise such as walking or stationary cycling, with the goal of increasing heart rate.

Stage 3. Sport-specific exercise such as running or skating, with the goal of additional movement.

Stage 4. Non-contact training drills, with an introduction of resistance training and more intense exercise, with the goal of maintaining coordination and multitasking.

Stage 5. Full contact practice, which is allowed following medical clearance, with a goal of a safety-first practice that helps foster confidence while coaches and clinicians assess functional skills.

Stage 6. Unrestricted return to sport.

because of prolonged rest, or not addressing persistent symptoms in concussion, can lead to prolonged neuropsychiatric disability—a concept that will be further explored in the upcoming chapters.

TAKE-HOME POINTS

- Return-to-play protocols have evolved over the years, and now include an unqualified recommendation of no return to play the same day as a concussion.
- Physical and cognitive rest are the cornerstone of recovery, but are no longer recommended beyond 24–48 hours.
- Premature return to play may increase the risk of subsequent concussion with the first 10 days following concussion.
- Prolonged cocoon therapy may increase the risk of prolonged neuropsychiatric symptoms.
- Return to play calls for a stepwise increase in activity, with at least 24 hours of successful activity at any stage before progressing to the next stage.

Further Reading

1) Broglio SP. Return to play following sports-related concussion. In Hainline B, Stern RA (Eds.), *Sports Neurology*, San Diego: Elsevier BV, 2018, pp 193–198.

2) McCrory P, Meeuwisse W, Dvorak J, et al. Consensus statement on concussion in sport—the 5th international conference on concussion in sport held in Berlin, October 2016. *Br J Sports Med* 2017;51:838–847.

3) Harmon KG, Clugston JR, Dec K, et al. American Medical Society for Sports Medicine position statement on concussion in sport. *Br J Sports Med* 2019;53:213–225.

4) Gibson S, Nigrovic LE, O'Brien M, et al. The effect of recommending cognitive rest on recovery from sport-related concussion. *Brain Inj* 2013;27:839–842.

10 Objective Biomarkers and Concussion (My white matter tracts are abnormal—what does that mean?)

A 21-year-old college senior presented with persistent symptoms after she sustained a concussion during a soccer game six months earlier. She had collided with another player while attempting a header on a free kick. She was off balance after the collision and was immediately removed from play, but there were no other symptoms to warrant referral to an Emergency Department. She was managed by her athletic trainer and a local neurologist, who prescribed two weeks of strict rest. Results of a routine brain magnetic resonance imaging (MRI) were normal. But when she attempted to return to school and engage in light exercise, her symptoms worsened; she then was placed back on strict rest. Her neurologist subsequently ordered a "specialized" brain MRI, including diffusion tensor imaging (DTI); this scan revealed increased fractional anisotropy in her white matter tracts. She was told that she had brain damage, should retire from sport, and should receive permanent accommodations in school.

What do you do now?

OBJECTIVE BIOMARKERS AND CONCUSSION

When an individual arrives at the emergency department with complaints of chest pain, and there is a suspected myocardial infarction, several tests are done to objectively assess the situation. By contrast, there are no objective biomarkers to diagnose concussion, although promising studies in search of such tests are underway. In the meantime, concussion remains a clinical diagnosis primarily based on subjective symptoms. Inadequate normative data sets and inconsistent data acquisition hamper current development of imaging biomarkers. Furthermore, highly selected populations, inconsistent definitions of concussion, and inadequate controls make the results of biomarker studies impossible to generalize.

In this case, the patient was told that her abnormal brain MRI results were consistent with permanent brain injury, but her provider was relying on results of tests not yet validated for concussion. For example, earlier studies of the blood biomarker ubiquitin C-terminal hydrolase L1 (UCH-L1) and glial fibrillary acidic protein (GFAP) predicted cerebral hemorrhage demonstrated by brain CT scans in patients with head trauma, but we are far from conclusively identifying a new blood biomarker to predict concussion. Nonetheless, promising biomarkers are now being developed for neuroimaging, blood tests, and genetic testing.

Biomarkers can be grouped into acute markers of injury, subacute markers of injury, and chronic markers of injury. Neuroimaging studies are a promising approach to objectively document biomarkers for both acute concussion and concussion recovery (Table 10.1). A brain CT scan is not an objective biomarker of concussion, but can be used to rule out an intracranial bleed, a fractured skull, or other obvious brain injury. Routine brain MRI studies are also not sources of objective data for diagnosing concussion, since they are routinely normal in cases of suspected concussion.

Emerging neuroimaging biomarkers include the following:

- DTI allows a detailed assessment of the white matter tracts of the brain. White matter abnormalities are described as either an increase or decrease in fractional anisotropy, which measures the restriction of fluid flow in the brain. Some studies using DTI have reported increased fractional anisotropy and others decreased fractional

TABLE 10.1 **Advanced Neuroimaging Biomarkers Investigated to Date**

More Promising	Less Promising
Diffusion tensor imaging	Electroencephalogram (EEG)
Magnetic resonance spectroscopy	Functional MRI (fMRI)—task based and resting state
Quantitative EEG	Measures of cerebrovascular reactivity
Cerebral blood flow	Arterial spin labeling
	Functional near-infrared spectroscopy
	Susceptibility weighted imaging

    anisotropy up to six months following injury. The reasons for these conflicting results need to be elucidated.

   · Functional brain MRI (fMRI) can determine functions of the brain when specific tasks are performed. However, this modality does not yield sufficiently high-quality data to determine the significance of abnormalities on fMRI following concussion.

   · Magnetic resonance spectroscopy has revealed a reduction in N-acetyl aspartate following concussion, with subsequent recovery by 30 days. However, some studies reveal chronic changes in N-acetyl aspartate following concussion, so the significance of these findings is not clear.

   · MRI studies can assess cerebral blood flow following concussion, and typically cerebral blood flow is decreased in the acute stages after injury. Cerebral blood flow can also increase following concussion, but the timeline for changes in cerebral blood flow remains unclear.

A landmark study from the NCAA–Department of Defense Concussion Assessment, Research and Educational Consortium (CARE) demonstrated that various MRI biomarkers can be reliably assessed within subjects, between sites, and between subjects at a site, given proper harmonization of protocols and equipment. These results are a major advance toward the goal of identifying objective neuroimaging biomarkers of concussion.

TABLE 10.2 **Advanced Fluid Biomarkers Investigated to Date**

More Promising	Less Promising
Alpha-amino-3-hydroxy-5-methyl-4-isoxazoleproprionic acid receptor peptide	Neuron-specific enolase
S100 calcium binding protein	Visinin-like protein-1
Neurofilament light	Total tau
Marinobufagenin	Salivary cortisol
Plasma soluble cellular prion protein	
Glial fibrillary acidic protein	
Calpain-derived alpha-II spectrin N-terminal fragment	
Ubiquitin C-terminal hydrolase L1	
Metabolomics profiling	
Early: tau-a, tau-c, SNTF, quinolinic acid, prolactin	
Chronic decreased amyloid-beta-42 in cerebrospinal fluid	

Many fluid biomarkers for concussion are now being tested, both in plasma and serum (Table 10.2), and there are preliminary studies of salivary biomarkers underway. Fluid biomarkers may measure necrosis, axonal injury, glial damage, apoptosis, demyelination, microglia response, or chronic inflammatory responses to blood vessels and neurons. To date, there are no objective fluid biomarkers that can either diagnose concussion or provide a prognosis for recovery. However, several emerging biomarkers are being explored (e.g., UCH-L1 and GFAP, mentioned earlier). Since such biomarkers could predict more severe head injury with associated brain hemorrhage, the hope is that they—or other biomarkers—can also predict concussion.

Genetic testing studies are emerging; these include examinations of brain modulation of the dose of injury, brain modulation of repair and resilience, and interactions between genetics and other behaviors (Table 10.3).

TABLE 10.3 **Genetic Biomarkers Investigated to Date**

Gene Expression	Genetic Variation Predicting Worse Outcome
Inflammatory pathway genes	Long variable tandem repeat alleles in the promoter of GRIN2A (NMDA glutamate receptor subunit)
Hypothalamic-adrenal-pituitary axis genes	Apolipoprotein E e4 allele
	Rs74174284 polymorphism in promoter of SLC17A7 C allele

Although a genetic profile could someday be developed to help athletes make informed decisions about participation in contact/collision sports, such testing is not yet available.

Overall, however, all medical diagnoses are ultimately clinically based, and combine a careful history and physical exam with supporting objective tests. The field of concussion is evolving so that a combination of clinical profiles and objective tests will one day more reliably diagnose this condition and provide future prognostic indicators.

TAKE-HOME POINTS

- Studies of many biomarkers show potential for better understanding the degree of brain injury and expectations for recovery in patients with brain injury.
- No biomarkers currently have sufficient evidence to support their use in clinical practice for diagnosing concussion, predicting recovery, or quantifying the amount of damage in a specific individual.
- Inadequate normative data sets and inconsistently acquired data are current obstacles to development of imaging biomarkers.
- Highly selected populations, inconsistent definitions of concussion, and inadequate controls make the results of current biomarker studies impossible to generalize.

Further Reading

1) McCrea M, Meier T, Huber D, et al. Role of advanced neuroimaging, fluid biomarkers and genetic testing in the assessment of sport-related concussion: a systematic review. *Br J Sports Med* 2017;51:919–929.
2) Kaplan S, Belson K. Concussions can be detected with new blood test approved by F.D.A. *New York Times*, February 14, 2018.
3) Nencka AS, Meier TB, Wang Y, et al. Stability of MRI metrics in the advanced research core of the NCAA-DoD concussion assessment, research and education (CARE) consortium. *Brain Imaging Behav* 2018;12:1121–1140.

11 Managing Expectations Following Concussion (Steve was diagnosed with a "mild TBI" three weeks ago and was told to follow up)

Steve, a 31-year-old investment banker, was riding his bicycle to work three weeks ago when he collided with an open taxicab door. His head hit the ground and he immediately felt dazed and nauseated. Emergency Department results were unremarkable, and he was diagnosed with a "mild traumatic brain injury." He spent the rest of the day and the subsequent weekend resting at home in a dark, quiet room. Since returning to work, he has been overwhelmed by the office lights, computer screens, and the noise produced by his colleagues. He is experiencing intermittent headaches and nausea and feels his "brain is moving too slowly" to function at his previous level at work. He confides that his greatest fear is ending up like his brother who, at 35, suffered a severe traumatic brain injury in a motor vehicle collision and never resumed his work as an attorney due to persistent cognitive and emotional difficulties.

What do you do now?

MANAGING EXPECTATIONS FOLLOWING CONCUSSION

Diagnostic Terminology

While the terms "mild traumatic brain injury" (mTBI) and "concussion" are often used interchangeably in the literature and clinically, the most recent Veterans Affairs and Department of Defense practice guidelines recommend using the terms "concussion" or "history of mild TBI" when communicating with patients. The goal is to convey that this is a transient condition from which full recovery is expected. The guidelines recommend against referring to patients as "mTBI patients" or "patients with mTBI," since these terms imply persistent injury. The terms "brain damage" or "brain injury" may inadvertently reinforce patients' expectations of persistent deficits and secondarily contribute to worse outcomes, although how much this phenomenon—known as "diagnosis threat"—contributes to lasting post-concussive symptoms remains unclear. Multiple studies have reported underperformance on cognitive assessments in patients with mTBI/concussion when their history of brain injury was mentioned, compared to similar participants given more neutral instructions. In studies of healthy controls, subjects allocated greater recovery time, greater undesirability, and greater expectations of lasting symptoms in vignettes where mTBI (rather than concussion) was the diagnosis.

While the effects of diagnosis threat can be difficult to undo once they occur, evidence from the larger field of "stereotype threat" suggests that appealing to individuals' multiple social identities may provide an alternative means of conceptualizing the self that may reduce the effect of the stereotype. In this case, informing Steve that he is likely to have a good recovery because of his relative youth, high education, and milder injury (compared to his brother's) may reduce the possibility that mTBI becomes a defining feature of his identity.

Predictors of Persistent Post-Concussive Symptoms

Multiple pre-, peri-, and post-injury factors can contribute to the development of persistent post-concussive symptoms (Table 11.1). Older age, female sex, lower socioeconomic status, lower level of educational attainment or intellectual ability (lower "cognitive reserve"), preexisting neurologic

TABLE 11.1 **Risk Factors for Prolonged Post-Concussive Symptoms**

Pre-injury	· Older age
	· Female gender
	· Lower socioeconomic status
	· Lower "cognitive reserve"
	· Preexisting neurologic or psychiatric disorder
Peri-injury	· More severe acute symptoms
	· Psychologically traumatizing event
Post-injury	· Poor expectation of recovery
	· Tendency to attribute nonspecific symptoms to brain injury
	· Involvement in litigation

conditions, and pre-morbid psychiatric illness are all known risk factors for persistent post-concussive symptoms. More severe symptoms at acute presentation and greater psychological trauma related to the event (e.g., assault) are associated with poorer long-term outcomes. Poor expectations for recovery, tendency to attribute common symptoms (e.g., fatigue, irritability) to brain injury versus other causes, and involvement in litigation have been associated with persistent symptoms after injury.

Managing Expectations after Concussion

Early education and empowerment are crucial first-line interventions for reducing risk of persistent post-concussive symptoms, along with appropriate early symptomatic relief (Table 11.2). In one prospective study, patients given informational booklets outlining expected post-concussive symptoms and suggesting coping strategies one week after concussion reported fewer symptoms and less overall stress at three months than patients not given this early intervention. In another study, patients given focused telephone counseling soon after the injury showed similar improvements. However, a recent study demonstrated worse outcomes in patients given a focused "health education intervention" compared to standard care, suggesting that early symptom education in some patients may worsen symptoms. While more research is needed using standardized approaches to concussion

TABLE 11.2 **Best Practices for Preventing Persistent Post-Concussive Symptoms**

General approach	· Focus on promoting recovery and avoiding harm · Follow a patient-centered approach that validates symptoms and elicits patient beliefs about projected recovery while providing reassurance and motivation · Capitalize on patients' perceived strengths and emphasize positive prognostic indicators when possible
Diagnostic terminology	· Use "concussion" or "history of mild TBI," not "brain injury" or "brain damage" when communicating with patients · Avoid referring to "mTBI patients" or "patients with mTBI," as these terms imply continued presence of the injury
Early education	· Discuss expected symptoms and coping strategies · Emphasize transient nature of most symptoms and expectation of full recovery
Symptom assessment and management	· Address somatic symptoms (e.g., headache, dizziness) · Identify comorbid psychiatric symptoms—especially in patients who experienced traumatizing events—and treat appropriately · Be mindful of potential adverse effects of medications · Avoid formal neuropsychology testing within the first 30 days after injury

education, early education about expectations—combined with early identification and management of possible high-risk features—is recommended to prevent prolonged post-concussive symptoms.

Somatic, mood, and cognitive symptoms should be addressed in a timely fashion, with the goal of promoting recovery and avoiding harm through excessive interventions. Comprehensive neuropsychological testing within the first 30 days after concussion is not recommended, since most early cognitive symptoms will improve, and formal testing in the early post-concussion period may only reinforce maladaptive patient beliefs about cognitive impairment.

· Several pre-, peri-, and post-injury features are potential risk factors for prolonged post-concussive symptoms (see Table 11.1).

· Early education about concussion, symptom validation, and appropriate reassurance and empowerment are crucial first-line interventions for managing expectations about recovery and reducing risk of prolonged symptoms.

· Discussions with patients should emphasize strengths and expected recovery and should avoid terms such as "brain injury" or "brain damage."

Further Reading

1) Department of Veterans Affairs. VA/DoD Clinical practice guideline for the management of concussion-mild traumatic brain injury (version 2.0). 2016. https://www.healthquality.va.gov/guidelines/Rehab/mtbi/. Accessed May 6, 2019.

2) Fresson M, Dardenne B, Meulemans T. Influence of diagnosis threat and illness cognitions on the cognitive performance of people with acquired brain injury. *Neuropsychol Rehab* 2018 Feb;27:1–18.

3) Snell DL, Hay-Smith EJ, Surgenor LJ, et al. Examination of outcome after mild traumatic brain injury: the contribution of injury beliefs and Leventhal's Common Sense Model. *Neuropsychol Rehab* 2013;23:333–362.

4) Sussman E, Pendharkar AV, Ho AL, et al. Mild traumatic brain injury and concussion: terminology and classification. In Hainline B, Stern RA (Eds.), *Sports Neurology*, San Diego: Elsevier BV, 2018, pp 21–24.

PART II

Manifestations and Management of Persistent Symptoms Following Concussion

12 Post-Concussion Syndrome (I feel like I'm in a black hole)

A 26-year-old male football player was injured during a kickoff play. He was one of the first players downfield, attempting to tackle the opponent who had received the football. He received a blindsided block, which led to a helmet-to-helmet collision with another player. Because of the collision, his right medial meniscus was torn, and he also suffered a concussion. He had immediate complaints of severe headache, dizziness, and considerable pain to his right knee. He was helped off the field and was evaluated in the locker room. He required surgical repair of the meniscus tear, and he never fully recovered from the surgery, nor did he ever return to football. He developed refractory knee pain, and was ultimately diagnosed with complex regional pain syndrome, type I. In addition, he developed refractory migraines, with associated anxiety, poor concentration, and diminished memory. He was diagnosed with post-concussion syndrome and was told there was nothing more to be done.

What do you do now?

POST-CONCUSSION SYNDROME

"Post-concussion syndrome" is a diagnostic term that assumes the presence of common influencers of delayed recovery. However, this diagnosis lacks clear consensus, and comprises a constellation of symptoms and signs not specific to concussion or brain injury. Indeed, emerging consensus is that post-concussion syndrome should no longer be used as a diagnostic term. In the fifth international consensus statement, the expert consensus is that "persistent symptoms" is the preferred term for individuals who do not follow the trajectory of normal clinical recovery. Further, "persistent symptoms" does not reflect a single pathophysiologic entity, but rather a constellation of nonspecific post-traumatic symptoms that may be linked to comorbid or cofounding factors.

Similarly, in the American Medical Society for Sports Medicine position statement on concussion, the authors describe clinical profiles or clinical domains that could justify more specific targeted treatment options. This is an emerging concept that does not necessarily represent clinical standards or norms. The position statement notes that individuals with persistent symptoms beyond the expected recovery time (> 2 weeks in adults, > 4 weeks in children) should be classified as having persistent post-concussive symptoms, not necessarily reflecting ongoing concussive injury to the brain.

The *Diagnostic and Statistical Manual of Mental Disorders* (5th edition; DSM-5) similarly no longer uses the term "post-concussion syndrome," but rather refers to "major or mild neurocognitive disorder: traumatic brain injury." Only the *International Classification of Diseases* (10th edition; ICD-10) manual still uses the term "post-concussion syndrome."

It is useful to group persistent post-concussion symptoms into broad domains of somatic, cognitive, or emotional complaints (Table 12.1). All may be influenced by a prior history of mental health disorders, neurologic conditions such as migraine and attention-deficit/hyperactivity disorder, genetics, age, and psychosocial influencers. The discerning clinician realizes that individuals who present with persistent post-concussion symptoms must be offered targeted treatment, often in a multidisciplinary setting.

In this case, this patient was told that there was nothing further to do. However, prominent influencers for this patient included his transition out of sport secondary to injury, development of nociplastic pain (mediated by

TABLE 12.1 **Domains of Persistent Post-Concussion Symptoms**

Somatic	Cognitive	Emotional
Headache	Decreased concentration	Irritability
Dizziness	Decreased attention	Anxiety
Fatigue	Decreased memory	Depression
Insomnia	Decreased processing speed	Emotional lability
Photo-phonophobia		
Pain		

psychosocial influencers), and clinical depression, all of which should be addressed. The core component of managing individuals with persistent post-concussion symptoms is psychoeducation. The main goal is to provide a framework for understanding the underlying condition, with a concrete action plan for successful management.

TAKE-HOME POINTS

· "Post-concussion syndrome" is no longer an accepted medical term.
· Post-concussion syndrome assumes a unified pathophysiology but is nonspecific.
· Individuals with persistent post-concussion symptoms should be assessed for their specific symptoms, and it should not be assumed that such symptoms are related to prolonged brain injury.
· Psychoeducation is the foundation of managing patients with persistent post-concussion symptoms.

Further Reading

1) Dwyer B, Katz DI. Postconcussion syndrome. In Hainline B, Stern RA (Eds.), *Sports Neurology*, San Diego: Elsevier BV, 2018, pp 163–178.

2) McCrory P, Meeuwisse W, Dvorak J, et al. Consensus statement on concussion in sport—the 5th international conference on concussion in sport held in Berlin, October 2016. *Br J Sports Med* 2017;51:838–847.

3) Harmon KG, Clugston JR, Dec K, et al. American Medical Society for Sports Medicine position statement on concussion in sport. *Br J Sports Med* 2019;53:213–225.

13 Sleep Disorder Following Concussion
(I feel constantly fatigued and have difficulty falling asleep)

A 32-year-old woman on a ski slope was struck from behind by another skier. She was upended, struck the back of her head, and tumbled down the hill. She lost consciousness briefly, and had difficulty standing up because of loss of equilibrium and severe headache. She was escorted down the hill on a sled, evaluated, and diagnosed with concussion. She did not ski for the rest of her trip, and returned home uneventfully. However, since then she has had persistent fatigue and difficulty falling asleep, and has begun to develop symptoms of depression. She has not returned to full exercise, and three months following this event, feels that her quality of life has been extremely poor.

What do you do now?

SLEEP DISORDER FOLLOWING CONCUSSION

Sleep disorders are under-diagnosed and under-managed in general, and are often under-recognized as a prominent cause of persistent symptoms following concussion. However, sleep disorder is one of many conditions now recognized as a contributor to persistent symptoms following concussion. Indeed, sleep and concussion are bidirectional influencers: individuals who develop sleep disorder following concussion are much more likely to develop prolonged, persistent symptoms, and prolonged, persistent post-concussion symptoms can trigger a sleep disorder.

Independent of concussion, sleep disorders increase the likelihood of developing mental health symptoms and disorders, decrease athletic performance, and decrease quality of life. Further, restorative sleep plays an important role in the glymphatic system, which may also aid recovery following concussion.

Sleep disorders are divided into primary sleep disorders (e.g., obstructive and central sleep apnea, narcolepsy, restless leg syndrome) and secondary sleep disorders (e.g., pain, depression, substance use disorder, and post-traumatic stress disorder). Individuals who present with persistent concussion symptoms should undergo a sleep assessment. This should begin with a basic clinical interview, which includes assessing for difficulty in falling asleep, frequent nighttime awakening, feeling exhausted upon awakening, and snoring. A sleep diary is often helpful in this regard. To further confirm a sleep disorder, questionnaires to capture self-reported symptoms such as those noted in Table 13.1 are useful. For protracted cases, polysomnography is recommended.

There is scant literature on effective intervention for sleep disorder following concussion. Table 13.2 provides an overview of managing sleep disorder among athletes, which can be extrapolated to managing sleep disorder after concussion. Importantly, a proper diagnosis guides treatment. For example, circadian dysregulation—a misalignment between the individual sleep-wake pattern and desired pattern—is common in athletes who travel. Adjustments to the training cycle and proper adaptations are keys to reducing the effects of circadian dysregulation. Sleep apnea may be particularly common among football players and may be exacerbated following concussion. Obstructive sleep apnea should be addressed through

TABLE 13.1 **Questionnaires for Self-Reported Sleep Disorder**

Insomnia Severity Index (for suspected insomnia)

Pittsburgh Sleep Quality Index (for suspected insomnia)

Epworth Sleepiness Scale (for daytime sleepiness)

Stanford Sleepiness Scale (for daytime sleepiness)

Morningness-Eveningness Questionnaire (for suspected circadian rhythm disorder)

Sleep Timing Questionnaire (for suspected circadian rhythm disorder)

any combination of weight loss, positive pressure airway devices, or surgery as needed. Nonpharmacologic treatments for sleep disorders should be the mainstay of treatment (except for well-documented obstructive sleep apnea), and the gold standard is cognitive behavioral therapy for insomnia (CBTI). CBTI is also effective for treating common comorbidities of sleep disorders such as persistent pain. Melatonin is the best-studied sleep aid in athletes, although its effectiveness following concussion has not been well documented. Establishing healthy sleep hygiene, coupled with progressive aerobic exercise, are also effective strategies to address sleep disorder following concussion.

TABLE 13.2 **Sleep Disorder Management**

Condition	Recommendations
Obstructive sleep apnea	Weight loss; positive airway pressure devices; surgery if indicated
Insomnia	Cognitive behavioral therapy for insomnia; sleep hygiene and aerobic exercise; trial of melatonin
Secondary to mental health symptoms or disorder	Cognitive behavioral therapy for insomnia; treatment of underlying mood disorder
Restless-leg syndrome	Dopamine agonists; gabapentin
Circadian rhythm disorder	Adjustment of training schedule and adaptation; sleep hygiene; trial of melatonin

- Sleep disorder is common in athletes and is a risk factor for mental health symptoms and disorders and diminished athletic performance.
- Sleep disorder is a risk factor for prolonged, persistent post-concussion symptoms.
- Prolonged, persistent post-concussion symptoms may kindle the development of sleep disorder.
- For athletes who present with persistent post-concussion symptoms, a thorough history of sleep disorder should be taken, including a sleep diary, a sleep screening questionnaire as needed, and polysomnography if appropriate.
- Management of sleep disorder depends on the underlying diagnosis. Sound nonpharmacologic strategies include cognitive behavioral therapy for insomnia and sleep hygiene, coupled with aerobic exercise.

Further Reading

1) Morse AM, Kothare SV. Sleep disorders and concussion. In Hainline B, Stern RA (Eds.), *Sports Neurology*, San Diego: Elsevier BV, 2018, pp 127–134.

2) Reardon CL, Hainline B, Aron CM, et al. International Olympic Committee consensus statement on mental health in elite athletes. *Br J Sports Med* 2019;53:667–699.

3) Rao V, McCann U, Han D, et al. Does acute TBI-related sleep disturbance predict subsequent neuropsychiatric disturbances? *Brain Inj* 2014;28:20–26.

4) Fogelberg DJ, Hoffman JM, Dikmen S, et al. Association of sleep and co-occurring psychological conditions at 1 year after traumatic brain injury. *Arch Phys Med Rehabil* 2010;92:1313–1318.

14 Migraine and Other Headache Disorders Following Concussion (My concussion caused severe headaches that won't go away)

An 18-year-old female rugby player developed concussion following a head-to-head collision. She felt dazed after the impact, and developed severe, global headache and associated neck pain. She had a prior history of well-controlled migraines that occurred about every two months and responded well to triptan medication. Following this injury, her headaches were somewhat similar to migraine, but became much more severe, with daily headache and superimposed fluctuations of daily, severe headache with associated photo- and phonophobia. She was treated with prolonged rest and told that her headaches were a manifestation of concussion. She was advised against taking triptan medication for this reason.

What do you do now?

MIGRAINE AND OTHER HEADACHE DISORDERS
FOLLOWING CONCUSSION

Headache is the most common manifestation of concussion. In many athletes, headache is the only manifestation of concussion, which has raised the question of whether a singular symptom such as headache is sufficient to diagnose concussion. This question remains unresolved, although prudence dictates that acute, post-traumatic headache should be managed as concussion until proven otherwise. Prolonged post-traumatic headache, without other concussion-related symptoms, is most likely a persistent symptom that needs to be addressed. That said, the complex relationships among headache, migraine, and concussion are not well understood.

About 24% of collegiate athletes self-report migraine, and an additional 25% self-report a history of sinus headache, which suggests that the true incidence of migraine may be under-diagnosed in this population. Emerging information indicates that a history of migraine predisposes to prolonged post-concussion symptoms. This predisposition may be related to an underlying pathophysiologic similarity between migraine and concussion, in that both manifest with electrical spreading waves of depression.

Individuals who present with persistent post-concussion headache should be assessed for a primary versus secondary headache disorder. Migraine is a primary headache disorder that can be exacerbated by concussion. By contrast, post-traumatic headache is a secondary headache disorder and can be differentiated into post-traumatic migraine, post-traumatic tension-type headache, post-traumatic cervicalgia, and post-traumatic headache nonspecified (distinguished from migraine). These distinctions are not straightforward and often are nuanced, as post-traumatic headache and migraine share similar pathophysiologic pathways and are often expressed in phenotypically similar ways. The term "persistent post-traumatic headache" is used to describe headache symptoms that persist 90 days or more following concussion.

Migraine and other post-traumatic headache disorders may also manifest with comorbid conditions such as sleep disorder, depression, anxiety, and cervicalgia. Regarding the latter condition, migraine frequently presents with nuchal pain, and occipital triggers can exacerbate migraine. This is especially important in concussion, since the impulsive forces that lead to concussion commonly cause violent whiplash-type movements of the neck.

No prospective studies provide clear guidance for patients with post-traumatic migraine or post-traumatic headache. Box 14.1 provides a list of recommended strategies. While no strategies have been proven, the discerning clinician understands that misdiagnosing post-traumatic migraine/post-traumatic headache as ongoing concussion can substantially limit an athlete's ability to return to play and considerably reduce his or her quality of life. On the other hand, the clinician must also discern when headache is a primary manifestation of concussion, and therefore not clear the athlete to return to play prematurely. Ultimately, if headache is the primary manifestation following concussion, then it should be addressed in a deliberate manner.

BOX 14.1. **Recommended Strategies for Management of Post-Traumatic Headache/Migraine**

Differentiate primary from secondary headache disorder.
  Search for treatable comorbid conditions such as sleep disorder, depression, and anxiety.
  Search for cervicalgia and other mechanical triggers of headache.
  Begin a deliberate approach to treatment that includes the following:

Nonpharmacologic Strategies	Pharmacologic/Injection Strategies
Cognitive behavioral therapy	Nonsteroidal anti-inflammatory drugs
Mindfulness	Triptan medications
Aerobic exercise	Antidepressants for mental health symptoms and disorders
	Prophylactic (antidepressants, anticonvulsants, etc.)
	Therapeutic injections (facet, occipital, sphenopalatine ganglion, or other branch nerve blocks)

· Athletes with migraine may be more predisposed to persistent post-concussion symptoms.

· Post-traumatic migraine and post-traumatic headache are common following concussion and share similar pathophysiologic mechanisms with concussion.

· It is important to distinguish post-traumatic headache/migraine from concussion.

  · Not recognizing post-traumatic headache/migraine as a manifestation of concussion can lead to premature return to play.

  · Not recognizing post-traumatic headache/migraine as a persistent symptom of concussion can lead to prolonged decrease in quality of life and delayed return-to-play options for the athlete.

  · There is scant evidence of any effective treatment for post-traumatic headache/migraine, but the discerning clinician should take a deliberate approach to addressing this matter.

Further Reading

1) Seifert T. The relationship of migraine and other headache disorders to concussion. In Hainline B, Stern RA (Eds.), *Sports Neurology*, San Diego: Elsevier BV, 2018, pp 119–126.

2) Seifert T, Sufrinko A, Cowan R, et al. Comprehensive headache experience in collegiate student athletes: an initial report from the NCAA headache task force. *Headache* 2017;57:877–886.

3) Echner JT, Seifert T, Pescovitz A, et al. Is migraine headache associated with concussion in athletes? A case-control study. *Clin J Sport Med* 2017;27:266–270.

15 Depression Following Concussion (I feel very depressed and lonely since my concussion)

A 20-year-old beach volleyball player presented with complaints of suicidal ideation. Six months earlier, she suffered a concussion while diving for the ball and colliding with her teammate. She immediately felt dizzy, and had complaints of neck pain and disequilibrium. She missed the rest of the season and underwent treatments for persistent neck pain and disequilibrium. She lost contact with her team, and was not asked to attend practices. She was a non-scholarship athlete and was not invited for team tryouts the next year. She felt increasingly isolated, developed increasing difficulty falling asleep at night, lost interest in food, and became increasingly withdrawn. She began to ruminate about death but did not have an active suicide plan.

What do you do now?

DEPRESSION FOLLOWING CONCUSSION

Depressive symptoms are common following concussion. Feeling slowed down, sad, more emotional, and having low energy are all commonly described post-concussive symptoms. Most patients recover from such symptoms within two weeks. However, some have persistent depressive symptoms, and some develop major depressive disorder. It is critical to differentiate depressive symptoms from a major depressive disorder. The DSM-5 criteria for major depressive disorder are noted in Table 15.1.

Transition out of sport is a risk factor for depression. Being part of a team, including team social activities, offers protective effects from depression symptoms. Similarly, exercise facilitates pathways that protect against depression. Thus, athletes who are forced to transition out of sport may be at higher risk for developing major depression disorder. Importantly, concussion alone is not a risk factor for suicide.

It is critical to differentiate depression symptoms, major depressive disorder, and prolonged brain injury. Individuals with persistent post-concussion depression often believe that they have developed a chronic

---

TABLE 15.1 **DSM-5 Diagnostic Criteria for a Major Depressive Episode**

At least 5 symptoms must be present for at least 2 weeks (at least 1 of the symptoms must be depressed mood, or decreased interest or pleasure):

· Depressed mood or (in children) irritable most of the day, nearly every day, as indicated by either subjective report (e.g., feels sad or empty) or observation made by others (e.g., appears tearful)	· Decreased interest or pleasure in most activities, most of each day
· Significant weight change or change in appetite	· Insomnia or hypersomnia
· Change in activity: psychomotor agitation or retardation	· Fatigue or loss of energy
· Feelings of worthlessness or excessive or inappropriate guilt	· Diminished ability to think or concentrate, or indecisiveness
· Recurrent thoughts of death or suicide	

TABLE 15.2 **Nonpharmacologic and Pharmacologic Management Considerations for Persistent Symptoms of Depression**

Nonpharmacologic	Pharmacologic
Psychoeducation	Bupropion
Psychotherapy, including cognitive behavioral therapy	Selective serotonin reuptake inhibitors
Exercise	Serotonin and norepinephrine reuptake inhibitors
Foster team activity	Tricyclic antidepressants; mirtazapine

brain injury and further believe they may be at risk for neural degeneration, when in fact addressing depressive symptoms or major depressive disorder may lead to resolution of the post-concussion persistent symptoms.

The discerning clinician must assess for all influencers of depression and must differentiate between depressive symptoms, major depressive disorder, and brain injury. Once this is done, the clinician should provide a foundation for management through psychoeducation. Other core principles of management include a combination of nonpharmacologic strategies, coupled with pharmacologic strategies when needed (Table 15.2). Of note, no prospective studies have demonstrated effective pharmacologic strategies for depression following concussion.

TAKE-HOME POINTS

· Depressive symptoms are common following concussion.
· It is important to differentiate depressive symptoms from major depressive disorder.
· Persistent symptoms of depression must be differentiated from brain injury.
· Concussion alone is not a risk factor for suicide.
· Management of persistent depression following concussion should include nonpharmacologic strategies, with pharmacologic strategies as needed.

Further Reading

1) McAllister TW, Wall R. Neuropsychiatry of sport-related concussion. In Hainline B, Stern RA (Eds.), *Sports Neurology*, San Diego: Elsevier BV, 2018, pp 153–162.

2) American Psychiatric Association. *Diagnostic and Statistical Manual of Mental Disorders (DSM-5)*. Washington, DC: American Psychiatric Publishing, 2013.

3) Vargas G, Rabinowitz A, Meyer J, et al. Predictors and prevalence of postconcussion depression symptoms in collegiate athletes. *J Athl Train* 2015;50:250–255.

16 Anxiety Following Concussion (I feel like I'm jumping out of my skin)

A 33-year-old female marathon runner presented with symptoms of severe anxiety and flashbacks. While training for the New York City Marathon in Central Park, she was attacked by two men and forced to the ground. Although she freed herself, she struck her head forcefully against the pavement. She has a poor memory of the event, and the assailants were never identified. Thereafter, she had a constellation of symptoms including headache, anxiety, dizziness, forgetfulness, and insomnia. She was diagnosed with concussion and was advised to discontinue running and to rest for the next two weeks. She ended her marathon training following this episode, and stopped running altogether. After two weeks of considerably restricted activity, her symptoms became worse. A neurologist advised that she was still suffering from concussion, and should continue to rest. Three months later, she remained symptomatic, with increasing symptoms of anxiety and intrusive flashbacks to the assault.

What do you do now?

ANXIETY FOLLOWING CONCUSSION

Symptoms of anxiety are common following concussion, including non-specific symptoms such as headache, dizziness, blurred vision, difficulty remembering, and feeling anxious. Additionally, after a concussion, individuals often complain of feeling irritable, having difficulty falling asleep, and feeling more emotional. As with depressive symptoms, most anxiety symptoms resolve within two weeks after a concussion. Also similar to depression, it is critical to differentiate anxiety disorder from post-concussion anxiety symptoms.

The inciting event of concussion may be so psychically charged that it triggers an acute stress or post-traumatic stress disorder. Both can occur after exposure to a traumatic event in which the individual perceives threat or serious injury; the response involves fear, helplessness, or horror. Ongoing symptoms can include depersonalization, detachment, flashbacks and distress on reminders of the event, coupled with avoidance of triggering stimuli, irritability, hypervigilance, restlessness, and impaired social/family activities. Acute stress disorder symptoms last for less than one month, whereas post-traumatic stress disorder is defined as exposure to trauma followed by at least one month of associated mental health symptoms. Thus, it is important to understand the individual's perception of the concussive injury, since the psychic/personal experience may be much more emotionally laden than what may be expected from obtaining a concussion history. Transition out of sport because of injury, marked reduction in exercise, and social isolation from teammates following concussion may further potentiate the development of persistent anxiety symptoms or anxiety disorder.

In this situation, the individual's concussion occurred during a psychically charged traumatic event. Further, the traumatic event was never resolved because the assailants were never identified, and the patient has only an incomplete memory of the events. This lack of resolution was complicated by her post-injury management, which included prolonged rest without other interventions. Emerging information tells us that prolonged rest is counterproductive following concussion, and can lead to increased post-concussive symptoms. When such symptoms increase, without a satisfactory diagnosis or psychoeducation in place, patients can feel hopeless, only worsening their situation.

TABLE 16.1 **Nonpharmacologic and Pharmacologic Management Considerations for Persistent Symptoms of Anxiety**

Nonpharmacologic	Pharmacologic
Psychoeducation	Selective serotonin reuptake inhibitors
Psychotherapy, including cognitive behavioral therapy, cognitive processing therapy, or prolonged exposure therapy	Benzodiazepines, short-acting anxiolytic medications as needed
Exercise	
Foster team activity	

The cornerstones of management for persistent anxiety symptoms or anxiety disorder include psychoeducation, psychotherapy, and pharmacologic therapy when needed (Table 16.1). The discerning clinician must differentiate anxiety-related symptomatology from brain injury.

TAKE-HOME POINTS

· Anxiety symptoms are common following concussion.
· Concussion injury may be psychically charged, which can potentiate acute anxiety disorder or post-traumatic stress disorder.
· The discerning clinician must differentiate between anxiety symptoms, anxiety disorder, and brain injury.
· Nonpharmacologic and pharmacologic therapies (as needed) should be instituted to treat persistent post-concussion anxiety and anxiety disorders.

Further Reading
1)   McAllister TW, Wall R. Neuropsychiatry of sport-related concussion. In Hainline B, Stern RA (Eds.), *Sports Neurology*, San Diego: Elsevier BV, 2018, pp 153–162.

2)   Dwyer B, Katz DI. Postconcussion syndrome. In Hainline B, Stern RA (Eds.), *Sports Neurology*, San Diego: Elsevier BV, 2018, pp 163–178.
3)   Soble JR, Silva MA, Vanderploeg RD, et al. Normative data for the neurobehavioral symptom inventory (NSI) and post-concussion symptom profiles among TBI, PTSD, and nonclinical samples. *Clin Neuropsych* 2014;28:614–632.

17 Emotional Dysregulation Following Concussion (Sarah has had mood swings since her concussion)

A 28-year-old volleyball player sustained a concussion when her head collided with the net pole. She felt dizzy and "saw stars" immediately, and sat out the rest of the game. One week later she was evaluated for persistent headaches, low mood, anxiety, and irritability, and was prescribed nortriptyline. Her mood, anxiety, and headaches improved significantly, but she felt that the effect plateaued after several weeks and she began to note bothersome fluctuations in mood and affect. She became tearful over television commercials and would find herself laughing and crying inappropriately during minor arguments with her boyfriend. She felt despondent when it rained but jubilant during sunny weather. She noted that nortriptyline initially imparted a marked energy boost, but this effect plateaued within a week. She felt exhausted by her mood swings and embarrassed by her frequent crying and laughing.

What do you do now?

EMOTIONAL DYSREGULATION FOLLOWING CONCUSSION

Emotional dysregulation or dyscontrol—a tendency to display unpredictable and rapidly shifting emotions—is common and usually transient in the first weeks after a concussion. Emotional dysregulation can encompass three related disorders of affect encompassed by this term: pathologic laughing and crying (PLC), also often referred to as pseudobulbar affect; affective lability; and irritability (Table 17.1). Although post-concussion management often focuses on symptoms such as headache, poor concentration and memory, and balance issues, emotional dysregulation is an important post-concussion presentation that can impair quality of life. As with other post-concussion manifestations, it is important to manage the clinical profile early, and to reassure the individual that emotional dysregulation does not indicate long-term brain injury.

Pathologic Laughing and Crying

Pathologic laughing and crying refers to brief, stereotyped expressions of intense emotion triggered by relatively minor stimuli and

TABLE 17.1 **Subtypes of Post-Concussive Emotional Dysregulation**

Pathologic laughing and crying	· Brief, stereotyped expressions of intense emotion · Triggered by neutral or trivial stimuli · Disproportionate to, or incongruent with, subjective mood · Cannot be modulated voluntarily
Affective lability	· Brief expressions of intense emotion · Less stereotyped, variable in intensity · Triggered by personally meaningful stimuli that previously would induce a less intense emotional response · Can be modulated by voluntary control or distraction · May be a feature of comorbid mood disorder
Irritability	· Subjective experience of being easily annoyed or overt reaction to minor stressors with quick anger · May be a feature of comorbid mood disorder

experienced as either incongruent with, or disproportionate to, the subjective emotional state during or between these moments. The brevity of these episodes distinguishes them from more sustained disturbances of affect seen in mood disorders. Patients often report distress or embarrassment at their inability to control their moment-to-moment emotional expression. PLC is most common immediately after injury and, in most patients, resolves over several weeks. The Pathological Laughing and Crying Scale (PLACS), developed to evaluate patients recovering from strokes, has not been validated among those who have sustained a concussion but may be a useful tool for identifying and characterizing PLC and tracking improvement. Education about PLC can help patients and families to understand and cope with symptoms. When PLC persists, is distressing, and has not improved after psychoeducation, then pharmacotherapy is warranted (Table 17.2). Selective serotonin reuptake inhibitors and tricyclic antidepressants are the first-line choices.

TABLE 17.2 **Nonpharmacologic and Pharmacologic Management Considerations for Persistent Emotional Dysregulation after Concussion**

	Nonpharmacologic	Pharmacologic
Pathologic laughing and crying	· Psychoeducation	· Selective serotonin reuptake inhibitors · Tricyclic antidepressants · Dextromethorphan-quinidine in select cases
Affective lability	· Psychoeducation · Psychotherapy · Neuropsychological interventions targeting emotional regulation	· Selective serotonin reuptake inhibitors · Anticonvulsants
Irritability	· Psychoeducation · Psychotherapy; anger management training · Neuropsychological interventions targeting emotional regulation	· Selective serotonin reuptake inhibitors · Anticonvulsants · Buspirone

Affective Lability

Affective lability, also described as emotional lability or mood swings, is the tendency to experience intense emotion in response to personally meaningful stimuli or events that would have otherwise evoked a more measured emotional response. Similar to PLC, affective lability manifests as brief episodes of intense emotional expression, but unlike PLC, episodes are less stereotyped, tend to vary in intensity, and often can be modulated by voluntary control or distraction. While affective lability is common after concussion, it can also be a feature of major depressive or bipolar disorders, substance use disorders, or personality disorders. Thus, its presence after concussion warrants consideration of these possible comorbidities. In particular, emergence of affective lability during antidepressant treatment may signal an underlying bipolar disorder. Treatment involves nonpharmacologic rehabilitation strategies focused on strengthening emotional regulation, plus pharmacologic approaches when warranted (Table 17.2). The Center for Neurologic Study–Lability Scale (CNS-LS), while not validated among those with concussion, may be a useful tool for characterizing and tracking affective lability in patients with concussion.

Irritability

Irritability occurs frequently after concussion and is conceptualized as a disorder of emotional control, in which patients may seem easily annoyed by minor stressors or react overtly to such stressors with quick anger. Self-reported annoyance is greater in patients with concussion than in healthy controls and also exceeded family and caregiver reports, suggesting the potential to exacerbate symptoms if patients feel their difficulties are not adequately acknowledged by loved ones. Irritability and reduced information-processing ability after concussion are correlated, reinforcing the importance of evaluating for comorbid subtle cognitive difficulties in patients after a concussion. Irritability can also be a feature of comorbid psychiatric disorders, or may be related to substance use, pain, or medication adverse effects; if these issues are present, they should be addressed first. Psychotherapy and neuropsychological rehabilitation to strengthen emotional regulation and cognitive performance are first-line treatment strategies, with pharmacologic interventions reserved for severe or persistent irritability (Table 17.2).

TAKE-HOME POINTS

· Emotional dysregulation is common after concussion, is usually transient, and may manifest as PLC, affective lability, or irritability.

· Affective lability and irritability may be directly concussion-related, or may be features of comorbid psychiatric disorders such as major depression or bipolar disorder.

· Pharmacotherapy is first-line treatment for persistent PLC. For affective lability and irritability, non-pharmacologic strategies are frequently effective. Pharmacotherapy should be reserved for more persistent and severe symptoms.

Further Reading

1) Arciniegas DB, Wortzel HS. Emotional and behavioral dyscontrol after traumatic brain injury. *Psychiatr Clin North Am* 2014; 37:31–53.

2) Moore SR, Gresham LS, Bromberg MB, et al. A self report measure of affective lability. *J Neurol Neurosurg Psychiatry* 1997;63:89–93.

3) Yang CC, Huang SJ, Lin WC, et al. Divergent manifestations of irritability in patients with mild and moderate-to-severe traumatic brain injury: perspectives of awareness and neurocognitive correlates. *Brain Injury* 2013;27:1008–1015.

18 Concussion and Attention-Deficit/ Hyperactivity Disorder (My focus is so much worse since my concussion)

A 15-year-old male baseball player was struck in the head by a line drive. He was not wearing a helmet, and the baseball struck the left frontal region of his head. He fell to the ground and required assistance getting up, and appeared wobbly and uncoordinated. Post-injury evaluation revealed no evidence of a skull fracture, and a brain CT scan was negative. He did not return to team activities following this incident. The patient's past medical history is notable for attention-deficit/hyperactivity disorder (ADHD), for which he was taking a combination of long- and short-acting stimulant medications. His ADHD symptoms were under good control prior to this incident. But since then, he has had increasing difficulty in focusing, and his teachers have noted his poor concentration in school, with subsequent diminishing grades. Adjusting his dose of the stimulant medication did not improve his symptoms.

What do you do now?

CONCUSSION AND ATTENTION-DEFICIT/ HYPERACTIVITY DISORDER

ADHD is a common brain developmental disorder, with prevalence ranging from 2.5% to 7.2% of youth. The core features of ADHD are age-inappropriate inattention, hyperactivity/impulsivity causing dysfunction in multiple settings, or both. Interestingly, children with ADHD may be attracted to sport because of the positive reinforcing and attentional activating effects of physical activity. The "hyperfocus" traits that are common in ADHD, coupled with reactive and quick decision-making, may draw children to sports such as baseball and basketball, where such quick movements and decisions are a core requirement. This is despite the fact that other symptoms of ADHD, such as lack of focus and concentration, may negatively impact an athlete's performance.

It is unclear whether athletes with ADHD are more prone to developing concussion. College athletes with ADHD report a higher history of concussion than athletes without ADHD. In athletes without a history of concussion, those with ADHD report more baseline symptoms than athletes without ADHD. Thus, ADHD may confer a certain risk for developing concussion (perhaps from inattention or risk-taking behavior, or from a lowered brain threshold following an impulsive force), and concussion symptoms may be more severe in athletes with ADHD compared to those without ADHD. Thus, it is critical to know if athletes with concussion have a diagnosis of ADHD, as the recovery trajectory may be misunderstood otherwise.

There are no prospective studies regarding the management of athletes with ADHD who sustain a concussion. However, psychosocial interventions are too often underused in athletes with ADHD, yet they may be as effective as medications in managing this condition. Any psychosocial interventions may be considered an alternative or a supplement to medication. Neurofeedback and EEG biofeedback may also have clinical utility in managing persistent ADHD symptoms following concussion. As with other persistent post-concussion symptoms, the discerning clinician must differentiate between ADHD as a risk factor for concussion, prolonged symptoms because of ADHD, and brain injury. Treatment should not focus solely on medication adjustment, but should include psychoeducation and psychosocial intervention, as warranted. Importantly, exercise and return to sport are key components of ADHD management.

Whereas stimulants are not an approved treatment for persistent post-concussion symptoms, athletes who have been diagnosed with ADHD and who are taking stimulants as part of their treatment should not have the stimulant medication withdrawn following a concussion. Emerging evidence informs us that maintenance and/or adjustment of stimulant medication following a concussion is one important aspect of post-concussion management of athletes with ADHD.

TAKE-HOME POINTS

- Individuals with ADHD may be drawn to certain sports.
- Collegiate athletes with ADHD self-report a higher history of concussion than collegiate athletes without ADHD.
- Athletes with ADHD have higher symptom scores at baseline relative to non-ADHD athletes.
- Nonpharmacologic strategies, especially psychosocial interventions, should be considered when managing persistent symptoms of ADHD.
- Stimulants should not be withheld from athletes with ADHD who suffer a concussion.

Further Reading

1) Nelson LD, Guskiewicz KM, Marshall SW, et al. Multiple self-reported concussions are more prevalent in athletes with ADHD and learning disability. *Clin J Sports Med* 2016;26:120–127.

2) Alosco ML, Fedor AF, Gunstad J. Attention deficit hyperactivity disorder as a risk factor for concussions in NCAA division-I athletes. *Brain Inj* 2014;28:472–474.

3) Perrin AE, Jotwani VM. Addressing the unique issues of student athletes with ADHD. *J Fam Pract* 2014;63(5):E1–E9.

4) Stewman CG, Liebman C, Fink L, et al. Attention deficit hyperactivity disorder: unique considerations in athletes. *Sports Health* 2018;10(1):40–46.

19 Concussion and Vestibular Dysfunction (I feel like I'm constantly seasick)

A 24-year-old male pole vaulter struck his head upon landing following an attempted vault. He was immediately extremely dizzy and nauseated, and his gait upon standing was quite wobbly. He was diagnosed with concussion and was advised to observe three days of strict bed rest, but he continued to have severe dizziness. He did not have classic vertigo, but rather felt unsteady, and stated that he felt like he was constantly seasick. His symptoms worsened whenever he was in a confined space, such as an aisle of a grocery store. Each time that he tried to do low-grade aerobic exercise, his symptoms worsened. He never followed a stepwise return-to-play protocol because he could never get beyond the first stage of tolerating low-grade aerobic exercise. He sought varying opinions and was always told that he had either concussion or post-concussion syndrome, and was advised to continue to rest until he could tolerate low-grade aerobic exercise.

What do you do now?

CONCUSSION AND VESTIBULAR DYSFUNCTION

Vestibular dysfunction is common following sport-related concussion. Acute dizziness with concussion injury is a predictor of prolonged recovery. Further, untreated vestibular dysfunction is a predictor of persistent symptoms, and is commonly misdiagnosed as post-concussion syndrome. There is emerging evidence that early treatment of vestibular dysfunction through targeted vestibular rehabilitation is efficacious and facilitates early recovery. Conversely, when vestibular symptoms interfere with a graded return to play, recovery can be prolonged, and the athlete becomes unable to return to sport.

It is important to distinguish peripheral from central etiologies of vestibular dysfunction (Table 19.1). Peripheral mechanisms of vestibular dysfunction following concussion include the following: (1) *benign paroxysmal positional vertigo*, which is associated with classic vertigo upon sudden head movement, especially changing from sitting to supine, and which is easily diagnosed with the Dix Hallpike maneuver; (2) *semicircular canal dysfunction*, which similarly can lead to vertigo and can be diagnosed with caloric testing or the Head Impulse Test; (3) *otolith dysfunction* of the utricle or saccule, which can lead to symptoms of feeling as if the individual is being pushed or pulled, walking on a boat, or walking on pillows. It can be diagnosed with ocular vestibular evoked myogenic potentials and the subjective visual vertical test.

Central mechanisms of vestibular dysfunction are less well understood, and may coexist with migraine, central oculomotor dysfunction, and autonomic dysfunction. *White matter abnormalities* are more common in

TABLE 19.1 **Peripheral and Central Mechanisms of Vestibular Dysfunction**

Peripheral	Central
Benign paroxysmal positional vertigo	Central oculomotor dysfunction
Semicircular canal dysfunction	White matter abnormalities and interruption of vestibular pathways (cerebellum, midbrain, thalamus, vestibular nuclei, etc.)
Otolith dysfunction	Autonomic dysfunction

patients with central vestibular dysfunction and may be associated with interruption of key central vestibular pathways. *Vestibular migraine* is a subtype of migraine that may improve with specific migraine treatment. Complaints of lightheadedness may be secondary to *autonomic dysfunction* following concussion. Impaired vagal cardiac autonomic modulation plus abnormal blood pressure responses to rest and graded exercise have been described following concussion. There is emerging information that progressive aerobic exercise helps to restore autonomic function and shortens recovery time.

The most common screening tool for vestibular dysfunction following concussion is the Vestibular/Ocular Motor Screening (VOMS) assessment (Table 19.2). This test has been validated and is increasingly used as an effective screening tool for vestibular dysfunction, an important diagnostic tool for concussion, and a predictor of prolonged recovery following

TABLE 19.2 **Vestibular/Ocular Motor Screening Assessment**

VOMS Tool	VOMS Procedure
Baseline complaints	Note complaints and symptoms
Smooth pursuits	Smooth pursuits should be done slowly, both horizontally and vertically. Change in symptoms should be noted.
Saccades	Test saccades horizontally and vertically. Overshoot and undershoot are abnormal. Change in symptoms should be noted.
Near-point convergence	Bring small object toward nose to point of double vision. Measure distance and symptoms.
Vestibular-ocular reflex	Test this reflex horizontally and vertically. Move the head as the individual fixes gaze straight ahead on a non-moving target. Assess gaze stabilization and record symptoms.
Visual motion sensitivity	The individual holds both arms outstretched with thumb up, then rotates torso/shoulders and thumb together while maintaining gaze on thumb. Change in symptoms should be noted.

Note: A positive test is an increase in symptoms or abnormal eye movements.

concussion. The VOMS measures baseline symptoms, smooth pursuit, saccades, near-point convergence, vestibular ocular reflex test, and visual motion sensitivity.

The discerning clinician should not assume that complaints of dizziness are simply a natural consequence of concussion. When vestibular dysfunction is identified, vestibular rehabilitation should be initiated, based on the nature of the vestibular dysfunction. Prompt recognition of vestibular dysfunction as a clinical profile of concussion and a common cause of persistent post-concussion symptoms will aid those who have been misdiagnosed with post-concussion syndrome.

TAKE-HOME POINTS

- Vestibular dysfunction is common in concussion, both as a clinical profile and as a cause of persistent symptoms.
- The type of vestibular dysfunction should be identified early in concussion management.
- Vestibular rehabilitation should be initiated early in individuals who suffer with post-concussion vestibular dysfunction.
- Vestibular rehabilitation is emerging as effective management for post-concussion patients with vestibular dysfunction.

Further Reading

1) Mucha A, Fedor S, Demarco D. Vestibular dysfunction and concussion. In Hainline B, Stern RA (Eds.), *Sports Neurology*, San Diego, Elsevier BV, 2018, pp 135–144.

2) Anzalone AJ, Blueitt D, Case T, et al. A positive Vestibular/Ocular Motor Screening (VOMS) is associated with increased recovery time after sports-related concussion in youth and adolescent athletes. *Am J Sports Med* 2016;45:474–479.

3) Leddy JJ, Baker JG, Kozlowski K, et al. Reliability of a graded exercise test for assessing recovery from concussion. *Clin J Sport Med* 2011;21:89–94.

4) McDevitt J, Appiah-Kubi KO, Tierney R, et al. Vestibular and oculomotor assessments may increase accuracy of subacute concussion assessment. *Int J Sports Med* 2016;37:738–747.

20 Autonomic Dysfunction Following Concussion (My heart races every time I walk)

A 35-year-old physical education teacher presents with dizziness. Three months earlier, she was playing tag with the children in her school and struck her head on the monkey bars. She fell backward, striking her head on the ground. She immediately felt dizzy and developed a severe headache. She was sent home early from school that day and upon returning the next day she felt that her heart was racing, she began to sweat profusely, became ashen, and nearly lost consciousness. She was evaluated that day at an urgent care center and was diagnosed with concussion, post-traumatic headache, and anxiety. After four weeks of treatment, which included migraine medication, vestibular rehabilitation, and a no-exercise protocol, she felt better and returned to work. However, upon any exertion at work, she felt dizzy and perceived that her heart was racing. Further evaluation revealed symptomatic orthostatic hypotension and tachycardia with prolonged standing.

What do you do now?

AUTONOMIC DYSFUNCTION FOLLOWING CONCUSSION

Although autonomic dysfunction is more common after moderate or severe traumatic brain injury, it contributes to acute and persistent symptoms following concussion, and it may present in various ways (Table 20.1). Cerebral blood flow is altered after concussion in animal models, and there is increasing evidence of abnormal heart rate variability in acutely concussed patients. This variability reflects an abnormal balance between sympathetic and parasympathetic outflow. The central network of control of autonomic function is complex and widespread, including brain areas such as the amygdala, brain stem, hypothalamus, insula, and prefrontal cortex. Given this diffuse network, it is not surprising that autonomic dysfunction develops following concussion.

Autonomic dysfunction frequently presents with abnormal responses to orthostatic position changes. Immediately upon standing, 300–800 mL of blood redistributes to the lower extremities and splanchnic venous systems, which causes lower cardiac output. The body must compensate for this change via increased activity of the sympathetic nervous system through vasoconstriction, increased heart rate and cardiac stroke volume, and decreased activity of vagal tone. In patients with autonomic

TABLE 20.1 **Presentations of Autonomic Dysfunction Following Concussion**

Orthostatic Hypotension	Postural Orthostatic Tachycardia Syndrome	Buffalo Concussion Treadmill Test
Sustained blood pressure reduction of systolic by 20 mmHg or diastolic by 10 mmHg at 3 minutes after standing, or at 60° in head-up position on a tilt table	Sustained heart rate increment of greater than 30 bpm within 10 minutes of standing, or at 60° in head-up position on a tilt table (for those ages 12–90, heart rate increment should be 40 bpm)	Increase of symptoms by 3 points on a 10-point Likert scale before achieving normal goal heart rate for aerobic activity

dysfunction, mechanisms to compensate for these changes are impaired; they may complain of feeling lightheaded, "dizzy," or feeling that their heart is racing. Such symptoms may be misinterpreted as vestibular dysfunction or anxiety.

Postural orthostatic tachycardia syndrome (POTS) is characterized by a persistent abnormally elevated heart rate in response to orthostatic position changes. A more extreme version of autonomic dysfunction is orthostatic hypotension. This condition is characterized by an abnormal drop in blood pressure, with or without an abnormal increase in heart rate. Patients with central nervous system–mediated or "neurogenic" orthostatic hypotension are less likely to have elevated heart rate on standing than patients with non-neurogenic causes of orthostatic hypotension. Patients with orthostatic hypotension may similarly complain of feeling dizzy, lightheaded, or sensing that their heart is racing.

Patients with concussion may also present with neurally mediated (vasovagal) syncope, caused by decreased sympathetic tone and corresponding increased vagal tone. Precipitating factors for this type of syncope include increased intra-abdominal pressure through straining, pain, anxiety, hyperventilation, or heat exposure.

When evaluating patients with suspected autonomic dysfunction after a concussion, non-concussion-related causes must also be considered. These include dehydration, cortisol and thyroid abnormalities, medications (vasodilators, beta-agonists, vasodilators, or dopamine agonists), and cardiac arrythmia. Tricyclic antidepressants may be used for other post-concussion symptoms such as headache, irritability, and insomnia, but these medications can worsen or even trigger autonomic dysfunction.

The Buffalo Concussion Treadmill Test has been used to identify abnormal autonomic function in acutely concussed patients by assessing for increased concussion-related symptoms after sub-maximal levels of aerobic activity. This assessment has been demonstrated as a safe way to both diagnose and manage post-concussion patients with autonomic dysfunction. Other strategies for minimizing symptoms related to autonomic dysfunction are outlined in Table 20.2.

TABLE 20.2 **Nonpharmacologic and Pharmacologic Management Considerations for Autonomic Dysfunction after Concussion**

Nonpharmacologic	Pharmacologic
Gradual change in position, from lying to sitting and then sitting to standing	Midodrine
Compression stockings	Fludrocortisone
Abdominal binders	
Pool exercise	
Increased salt and water intake	
Adequate management of anxiety	
Sub-symptom threshold exercise program	

TAKE-HOME POINTS

· Autonomic dysfunction is common and often incompletely assessed after concussion.
· Autonomic dysfunction is commonly experienced as dizziness, lightheadedness, or perceiving a racing heart.
· Autonomic dysfunction can mimic vestibular dysfunction and anxiety.
· Management of autonomic dysfunction should maximize nonpharmacologic strategies before considering pharmacologic management.
· Early sub-symptom threshold aerobic exercise appears to speed recovery after concussion.

Further Reading

1) Freeman R, Wieling W, Axelrod FB, et al. Consensus statement on the definition of orthostatic hypotension, neurally mediated syncope and the postural tachycardia syndrome. *Clin Auton Res* 2011;21: 69.
2) Leddy JJ, Baker JG, Kozlowski K, et al. Reliability of a graded exercise test for assessing recovery from concussion. *Clin J Sport Med* 2011;21:89–94.

3) Leddy J, Hinds A, Miecznikowski J, Darling S, Matuszak J, Baker J, Picano J, Willer B. Safety and prognostic utility of provocative exercise testing in acutely concussed adolescents: a randomized trial. *Clin J Sport Med* 2018;28:13–20.

4) Leddy J, Wilber C, Willer B. Active recovery from concussion. *Curr Opin Neurol* 2018;31:681–686.

21 Concussion and Oculomotor Dysfunction (Every time I try to read I get a headache and feel dizzy)

A 16-year-old male complained of headaches and feeling dizzy each time he tried to read. He had sustained a concussion when his head was slammed into the mat while practicing judo. He developed immediate symptoms of dizziness and headache, and he complained of intermittent double vision. He returned to school one week after the event, and his schoolwork was modified. However, he has been unable to read since this event. Each time he tries to read, he has difficulty focusing, and he develops headache and feels dizzy. Because of persistent complaints, he underwent a brain MRI scan, which was normal. A routine optometry exam also was normal. Results of a neurologic exam were described as "non-focal."

What do you do now?

CONCUSSION AND OCULOMOTOR DYSFUNCTION

Since visual pathways comprise 50% of the brain, it makes sense that oculomotor dysfunction is common following concussion. However, it is frequently under-diagnosed and under-managed because a careful eye exam is often not performed following concussion. The pupillary light reflex is commonly done in a cursory manner. Smooth pursuits are carried out too quickly. Saccades are not accurately measured. Near-point convergence is often not performed. This has begun to change with emerging appreciation of the simplicity and predictability of the Visual/Oculomotor Motor Screening (VOMS) assessment, which was described in the previous chapter.

Table 21.1 provides common pitfalls of the oculomotor exam. If the oculomotor exam is performed carefully, it is more likely to reveal subtle or overt abnormalities in oculomotor function. Emerging sideline and office tools to measure oculomotor function are promising. The King-Devick test is a time-based measure of saccadic eye movements; when combined with the SCAT5, it helps to confirm the diagnosis of concussion. The Mobile Universal Lexicon Evaluation System (MULES) is an emerging tool that more comprehensively assesses saccadic eye movements, coupled with color vision testing and object identification.

Video-oculography provides a detailed computerized assessment of eye movements, but is not practical for sports medicine clinicians because of the personnel and infrastructure requirements. Eye movement tracking devices are undergoing assessment and are being widely marketed as

TABLE 21.1 **Common Pitfalls of the Oculomotor Exam**

Exam	Pitfall
Pupillary light reflex	Pupil size and response time not observed
Smooth pursuits	Performed too quickly, without attention to subtle saccadic breaks
Saccades	Overshoot and undershoot not carefully documented
Near-point convergence	Not performed, or distance of double vision not measured

effective diagnostic tools for concussion, but their efficacy has not yet been demonstrated.

Oculomotor abnormalities are both a common clinical profile of acute concussion, and a common cause of persistent post-concussive symptoms. Oculomotor dysfunction and vestibular dysfunction commonly coexist, so patients with dizziness should be assessed in detail for both oculomotor and vestibular abnormalities. Similarly, patients with complaints of headache, especially while reading, should be assessed for an oculomotor dysfunction.

Oculomotor rehabilitation is an emerging strategy for both acute and subacute management of oculomotor dysfunction post-concussion. Accordingly, early rehabilitation of oculomotor disorders may help to prevent central sensitization of such dysfunction. As one example, "pencil push-ups" are an easy-to-perform and validated treatment for convergence insufficiency.

TAKE-HOME POINTS

· Oculomotor dysfunction is common following concussion.
· Oculomotor dysfunction is part of the clinical profile of acute concussion and persistent post-concussion symptoms.
· Oculomotor abnormalities are under-diagnosed and under-managed following concussion.
· Oculomotor rehabilitation is an emerging strategy that should be used early in treatment of patients who present with post-concussion oculomotor dysfunction.

Further Reading

1) Debacker J, Venura R, Galetta S, et al. Neuro-ophthalmologic disorders following concussion. In Hainline B, Stern RA (Eds.), *Sports Neurology*, San Diego: Elsevier BV, 2018, pp 145–152.

2) Clugston JR, Chrisman SPD, Houck ZM, et al. King-Devick test time varies by testing modality. *Clin J Sport Med* 2018; doi: 10.1097/JSM.0000000000000691.

3) Hasanaj L, Thawani SP, Webb N, et al. Rapid number naming and quantitative eye movements may reflect contact sport exposure in a collegiate ice hockey cohort. *J Neuroophthalmol* 2017;38:24–29.

4) Cobbs L, Hasanaj, L, Amorapanth P, et al. Mobile Universal Lexicon Evaluation System (MULES) test: a new measure of rapid picture naming for concussion. *J Neurol Sci* 2017;372:393–398.

22 Concussion and Pituitary Dysfunction
(I have not a period in four months)

A 15-year-old girl presented with amenorrhea that had lasted for four months. Four months ago, she suffered her third concussion within a year while playing soccer. The concussion resulted from a collision with another player. She was able to return to school and to sport within three weeks after each concussion, but has not menstruated since the last concussion. She began menstruating at age 12 and previously had a regular monthly cycle. She had a healthy diet, with no evidence of disordered eating.

What do you do now?

CONCUSSION AND PITUITARY DYSFUNCTION

Endocrine abnormalities may be under-diagnosed and under-managed following concussion. Since 90% of the world literature on concussion refers to concussion in males, even less is known about endocrine dysfunction in female athletes with concussion. Because concussion may involve shearing forces to both the hypothalamus and pituitary, the hypothalamic-pituitary axis may be vulnerable following concussion and brain injury. Indeed, because the pituitary gland is situated within the sella turcica, its vasculature may be particularly susceptible to single or repetitive shearing forces.

The hypothalamic-pituitary axis is critical in the development of secondary sexual characteristics, bone development, neuroplasticity, myelination, neurogenesis, and the production of neurotrophic growth factors. Hypopituitarism could thus have a profoundly negative effect on normal adolescent development. Hypopituitarism also adversely impacts adults. Symptoms such as depression, loss of libido, lethargy, impaired concentration, and decreased problem-solving ability are all characteristics of hypopituitarism in adults.

The discerning clinician should have a low threshold for assessing the hypothalamic-pituitary axis in individuals with persistent symptoms consistent with hypopituitarism, or with overt symptomatology such as menstrual dysfunction. Box 22.1 lists ancillary tests that should be considered when hypopituitarism is suspected. Hopefully, future research will address this matter in more detail, since many individuals diagnosed with postconcussion syndrome may instead have hypopituitarism.

BOX 22.1. **Ancillary Blood Tests for Suspected Hypopituitarism**

Thyroid-stimulating hormone
Insulin-like growth factor
Adrenocorticotrophic hormone (ACTH)
Prolactin
Luteinizing hormone
Follicle-stimulating hormone
Growth hormone

· Because of their anatomic location, the hypothalamus and pituitary may be susceptible to shearing forces that are common in concussion.

· The hypothalamic-pituitary axis is critical in adolescent development and plays an important role in normal adult function.

· Hypopituitarism is likely under-diagnosed and under-managed following concussion.

· Clinicians should have a low threshold for evaluating the hypothalamic-pituitary axis in patients with persistent post-concussive symptoms, especially when such symptoms are consistent with hypopituitarism.

Further Reading

1) Snook ML, Henry LC, Sanfilippo JS, et al. Association of concussion with abnormal menstrual patterns in adolescent and young women. *JAMA Pediatr* 2017;171:879–886.

2) Bigler ED. Neuropsychology and clinical neuroscience of persistent post-concussion syndrome. *JINS* 2008;14:1–22.

3) Tanriverdi F, Unluhizarci K, Karaca Z, et al. Hypopituitarism due to sports related head trauma and the effects of growth hormone replacement in retired amateur boxers. *Pituitary* 2010;13:1111–114.

23 Women and Concussion (Julie has persistent symptoms after her concussion, but her brothers think she is just "being dramatic")

Julie, a 19-year-old college sophomore soccer player, sustained a concussion three months ago when she collided with another player while heading the ball. She saw "sparkles" briefly and experienced immediate tinnitus, vertigo, and nausea. She sat out the rest of the game. Since then, she has complained of persistent mild fatigue, lightheadedness, and difficulty concentrating. She has seen her primary care doctor twice for these symptoms and was told to "give it time." She felt well enough to return to playing soccer but remains anxious about her continued symptoms. Her two older brothers, both athletes with previous concussions, have recommended that she "just get over it" and have joked that she should "stop being such a girl." She feels that no one appreciates the severity of her symptoms and worries that "something may be really wrong" with her because she is not recovering as her brothers did.

What do you do now?

WOMEN AND CONCUSSION

Sex is a biological determination based on chromosomes that manifests as specific hormonal and anatomic attributes, while *gender* refers to features of behavior and identity expressed with regard to a set of social, cultural, and environmental norms. How sex and gender influence concussion has only recently begun to garner significant attention. Both sex-based and gender-normative factors may be responsible for differential outcomes after concussions in men and women.

Prevalence

Most studies of concussion in animals suggest that females are relatively protected, but data from human studies are more mixed. Women who play soccer, basketball, or baseball/softball have proportionally more concussions than their male counterparts. However, studies of ice hockey and lacrosse players have not shown consistent differences. Concussion-specific data are more limited for the general population; studies have tended to examine concussion in the context of traumatic brain injury (TBI) of all severities, but rates generally track with the overall trend toward increased prevalence of TBI in men. In military populations, where women are a fast-growing cohort, limited data suggest that they have rates of deployment-related concussion equivalent to men.

Injury Mechanisms

The reasons for increased vulnerability to concussion among female athletes are unclear. While injury mechanisms such as type of impact do not generally appear to differ significantly by sex, baseline differences in head size and neck strength may play a role, since women's heads may be being exposed to higher acceleration forces because their cervical muscle strength is relatively lower than men's. Emerging data suggest that injury mechanisms may differ in particular sports; e.g., male soccer players have more concussions while heading the ball because of head-to-head or elbow-to-head contact, whereas their female counterparts develop concussions during heading the ball from losing balance and striking their head on the turf. The implications of such data are not yet clear. At the cellular level, women's axons may be smaller with fewer microtubules than men's, placing them at greater likelihood of disruption when exposed to any given force. Women of childbearing age appear to have the worst outcomes, suggesting a possible role for sex hormones in the pathogenesis of concussion. One study demonstrated poorer outcomes for women injured during the luteal phase of the menstrual cycle compared to women injured during the follicular phase or those taking oral contraceptives. The authors surmise that abrupt progesterone withdrawal in the setting of hypothalamic-pituitary-gonadal axis dysfunction may hamper recovery after a concussion.

Post-Concussive Symptoms

After a concussion, women consistently report more post-concussive symptoms—whether among athlete, general, or military populations. Because of possible higher baseline rates of post-concussion-like symptoms in non-concussed women versus men, some have suggested that women may simply be more likely to experience symptoms of concussion in general. Anxiety sensitivity (a tendency to fear and overinterpret bodily sensations associated with anxiety) may be more common in women and has been proposed as a potential mediator of some reported differences in reports of post-concussive symptoms between men and women.

Cultural gender norms likely also influence symptom reporting. Female athletes demonstrate increased intention to report future concussive symptoms, but in both male and female athletes the degree of conformity to typical masculine norms (e.g., risk-taking and valuing winning) is associated with decreased likelihood of reporting symptoms and increased willingness to play while symptomatic. The circumstances surrounding the concussion may also play a role; for example, women are more likely to be victims of intimate partner violence (IPV), and brain injury is a common consequence of IPV. Exposure to IPV was itself associated with increased neurobehavioral symptom reporting in one study of female veterans. More research is needed in this area.

Recovery

Despite reporting greater post-concussive symptoms, women and men appear to recover at similar rates, with comparable numbers of days to return to activity. Some studies report decreased processing speed, slower reaction times, and increased likelihood of cognitive deficits in concussed women compared to men, while other studies have shown no difference. The most consistent finding appears to be some relative impairment in visual memory in concussed women versus men in the post-acute period. However, this difference has also been shown in healthy populations, highlighting the need for sex-specific normative data. When the cognitive impact of multiple concussions was examined, women outperformed men on visual memory measures and other cognitive tasks, suggesting that concussion severity may differ across the sexes and that this difference may have a cumulative effect. Premorbid ADHD and learning disability (both more common in men) also may influence post-concussive cognitive outcomes, although more research is needed in this area as well.

Overall, sex-based biological differences and culturally based gendered behavioral patterns likely both influence outcomes in concussion (Table 23.1). In this case, it is appropriate to validate Julie's experience and to

TABLE 23.1 **Concussion in Women**

Prevalence	· Higher rates of sport-related concussion · Lower rates of TBI more generally
Sex-based differences	· Relatively weaker neck strength may contribute to greater head acceleration on impact · Smaller neuronal axons with fewer microtubules may be more prone to injury · Phase of menstrual cycle at time of injury may play a role · Mechanism of injury may play a role
Gender-based/ sociocultural differences	· More likely to report symptoms · Degree of adherence to masculine norms in sports may influence symptom reporting and likelihood of continuing to play while symptomatic · More likely to be exposed to concussion in setting of intimate partner violence
Baseline symptom profiles	· More concussion-like symptoms at baseline · Relatively weaker visual memory · Relatively stronger verbal memory
Post-concussion outcomes	· Report greater number of symptoms · Relative impairment in visual memory · Similar rates of return to play/activities as men

reassure her that while her recovery trajectory may differ from her brothers', a good outcome is still expected. Not doing so may lead her to believe that her injury is being dismissed or has been misunderstood. This could lead to Julie focusing too much attention and emotional weight on the concussion and its residual symptoms as she attempts to make others understand her distress. Clinicians should be mindful of these differences, maintaining an open, nonjudgmental stance—both to validate the recovery trajectories of female patients if they differ from what were (until relatively recently) largely male data sets, and to allow male patients to report symptoms they might have otherwise hidden.

TAKE-HOME POINTS

· Women appear to be more prone to sport-related concussion than men.
· There are both sex-based and cultural gender-based differences in how men and women experience and describe concussion.
· While women report more concussion-like symptoms at baseline and consistently report more post-concussive symptoms than men, overall post-concussive outcomes are good for both sexes.

Further Reading

1) Bazarian J, Blyth B, Mookerjee S, et al. Sex differences in outcome after mild traumatic brain injury. *J Neurotrauma* 2010;27:527–539.
2) Kroshus E, Baugh C, Stein CJ, et al. Concussion reporting, sex, and conformity to traditional gender norms in young adults. *J Adolescence* 2017;54:110–119.
3) Merritt VC, Padgett CR, Jak AJ. A systematic review of sex differences in concussion outcome: what do we know? *Clin Neuropsychol* 2019 Jan;8:1–28.

24 Concussion and Cognitive Dysfunction
(Ever since I hit my head I have no short-term memory)

A 40-year-old man presented with complaints of short-term memory problems. Six months earlier, he fell off his mountain bike while going downhill. He was wearing a helmet and struck the side of his head on a large rock. He could not disengage from the pedals and tumbled forward for several meters following the head impact. He has a good memory of the event and recalls feeling that his life was in danger. He successfully navigated downhill for the rest of the trail and sought medical attention that day at an urgent care center. He was advised to go to the Emergency Department, where further evaluation revealed a negative brain CT scan, and he was diagnosed with concussion. Since the accident, he has been anxious and has had considerable difficulty with short-term memory. He has not returned to a regular exercise program.

What do you do now?

CONCUSSION AND COGNITIVE DYSFUNCTION

Cognitive dysfunction is common following concussion and usually resolves after several days. It has become commonplace to administer computerized cognitive tests as a baseline in high school, collegiate, and professional sport teams, although their value is not firmly established. Baseline cognitive tests are not available for most individuals with concussion, and cognition is assessed as part of a focused neurologic exam. Several cognitive domains are susceptible following concussion, including concentration, attention, processing speed, executive function, and short-term memory. These domains depend on a diffuse network of brain connectivity and are not localizable to specific brain regions.

Impaired cognition is a clinical profile of acute concussion and a hallmark of persistent post-concussion symptoms. It is extremely difficult to separate cognition from the many other profiles of concussion, including mental health symptoms and disorders, sleep impairment, vestibular and oculomotor dysfunction, hypopituitarism, and pain (including headache). Any of the profiles noted in Box 24.1 can interfere with normal cognition, and all must be considered when an individual presents with memory or other cognitive impairment after a concussion. Further, individuals with impaired cognition may secondarily develop anxiety symptoms or anxiety disorder because of the fear that they have permanent brain damage or a neurodegenerative condition.

The discerning clinician should assess all clinical domains of concussion when individuals present with cognitive impairment. Importantly, many individuals who have suffered concussion do not return to their baseline level of activity (exercise, social engagement) because they remain

---

BOX 24.1. **Clinical Profiles That Can Impair Cognitive Function**

Vestibular dysfunction
Fatigue and sleep impairment
Anxiety, depression, and other mental health symptoms and disorders
Headache, migraine, and other pain disorders
Oculomotor dysfunction
Hypopituitarism

symptomatic, and this further kindles a persistent cycle of inactivity-induced post-concussion symptoms. Thus, the clinical encounter should also include a careful psychosocial assessment.

When cognitive impairment persists despite management of other concussion clinical profiles and return to exercise, a referral to a neuropsychologist should be considered, rather than relying on a computerized test of cognition. A relatively new subspecialty, sports neuropsychology, applies the understanding of brain-behavior relationships to sport-related brain injury. Neuropsychologists, and in particular sports neuropsychologists, are uniquely qualified to tease apart the interrelationships of cognitive, behavioral, and psychosocial manifestations of possible brain injury. They are an integral part of multidisciplinary management of persistent post-concussion symptoms, and provide diagnoses and key management recommendations. For the individual described in the case-report, the neuropsychologist did document considerable short-term memory deficits in conjunction with untreated anxiety and fear since the accident. A comprehensive approach of cognitive behavioral therapy and return to exercise led to complete resolution of symptoms.

TAKE-HOME POINTS

· Cognitive complaints are common following concussion.
· Cognitive domains depend on a vast array of interconnected brain pathways.
· When assessing individuals with persistent cognitive dysfunction after a concussion, it is important to address all concussion clinical profiles.
· Sports neuropsychologists are uniquely qualified to evaluate individuals with persistent cognitive impairment following concussion.

Further Reading

1) Echemendia R, Gioia GA. The role of neuropsychologists in concussion evaluation and management. In Hainline B, Stern RA (Eds.), *Sports Neurology*, San Diego: Elsevier BV, 2018, pp 179–191.

2) Sports Neuropsychology Society. Sports neuropsychology: definition, qualifications, and training guidelines. http://www. sportsneuropsychologysociety.com/forms/SNS-Definition-Sports-Neuropsychologist.pdf.

3) Covassin T, Elbin RJ. The cognitive effects and decrements following concussion. *Open Access J Sports Med* 2010;1:55–61.

25 Neck Pain Following Concussion
(My neck is killing me ever since my car accident)

A 28-year-old woman presents with chronic neck pain. She dates this to five months earlier, when she suffered an inadvertent kick to the jaw while training in kickboxing. She recalls that her head moved violently in a posterior/rotational manner. She did not lose consciousness, but felt dazed and noticed considerable neck pain with some associated dizziness. She regained mental clarity within days, but has had persistent posterior neck pain, worsened with lateral rotation and flexion, without cervical radicular symptoms. She also has had intermittent, nonspecific dizziness. Further evaluation revealed unremarkable X-rays of the cervical spine (other than some lordotic straightening), and mild degenerative changes of C4–5 and C5–6 noted on an MRI scan of the cervical spine. Because of persistent symptoms, an epidural injection of corticosteroids into the cervical spine was recommended, which the patient refused.

What do you do now?

NECK PAIN FOLLOWING CONCUSSION

Although concussion often involves whiplash movements of the neck, there is a dearth of literature on diagnosis and management of cervicalgia following concussion. The mechanisms of concussion and cervical spine injury share many biomechanical similarities, and their clinical manifestations may overlap. The international consensus definition of concussion by the Concussion in Sport Group states that concussion is the result of a direct or indirect blow to the head and face, neck, or elsewhere on the body, with an impulsive force transmitted to the head. The neck is the epicenter of this impulsive force transmission.

During the impulsive forces of whiplash neck movement, cervical structures are vulnerable to stress and damage at their end range of motion. This includes cervical musculature, ligaments, zygapophysial joints, and intervertebral discs. The zygapophysial joints are a documented source of persistent posterior neck pain following concussion, especially with neck extension/rotation movements. Cervical muscles, especially the deep flexors and extensors, are subject to injury, with subsequent maladaptive response of spasm and limitation in neck range of motion, thereby setting up a circular response of ongoing spasm and limited neck motion. Such spasm can secondarily lead to cervicogenic headache.

Unrelated to pain, cervical spine trauma may be a source of faulty proprioceptive input to the vestibular nuclei from abnormal upper cervical spine efferents, manifesting as vestibular symptoms. Further, upper cervical sensory nerve roots converge with the trigeminal nucleus caudalis and may potentially activate the trigeminovascular system. Accordingly, the cervical spine should be carefully examined in all patients who present with neck pain, persistent vestibular symptoms, or cervicogenic headache after a concussion. Box 25.1 outlines the core features of the cervical spine exam.

Management of cervicalgia should be directed by the examination's findings. Unless there is a worrisome neurologic deficit, manual therapy should be a first choice. Even with zygapophysial joint irritation, manual release techniques and strengthening of the deep cervical muscles can often improve symptoms. The facet joints are not the primary source of movement, but rather the underpinning of the skeletal feasibility of movement. Physical therapy combined with isometric strengthening can promote

> **BOX 25.1. Core Features of the Cervical Spine Exam**
>
> Palpation of the posterior cervical spine and paraspinal muscles
> Active and passive neck range of motion
> > Forward flexion, backward extension, lateral flexion, rotation,
> > rotation combined with extension
> Resisted neck movement, including flexion, extension, lateral flexion,
> > and rotation
> Scapular and shoulder movement assessment
> Occipital groove and other trigger point assessment
> Visual motion sensitivity test (for patients with persistent dizziness)

intracortical inhibition and may relieve pain better than isotonic and eccentric exercises. There is emerging evidence that a combination of cervical spine manual therapy, neuromotor/sensorimotor training, and vestibular physiotherapy are very effective for patients who present with persistent symptoms of cervicalgia, dizziness, and cervicogenic headache after a concussion.

TAKE-HOME POINTS

- Cervicalgia and cervical spine injury may be common following concussion.
- The cervical spine should be carefully examined in individuals who have had a concussion.
- Cervicalgia and cervical spine injury following concussion may be a source of persistent symptoms.
- Cervicalgia with dizziness and cervicogenic headache should be managed with comprehensive physical therapy and vestibular therapy.

Future Reading

1)   Cheever K, Kawata K, Tierney R, et al. Cervical Injury assessments for concussion evaluation: a review. *J Athl Train* 2016;51(12): 1037–1044.

2) Morin M, Langevin P, Fait P. Cervical spine involvement in mild traumatic brain injury: a review. *J Sports Med* 2016; http://dx.doi.org/10.1155/2016/1590161.

3) Brandt T, Bronstein AM. Cervical vertigo. *J Neurol Neurosurg Psychiatry* 2001;71:8–12.

4) Schneider KJ, Meeuwisse WH, Nettel-Aguirre A, et al. Cervicovestibular rehabilitation in sport-related concussion: a randomized controlled trial. *Br J Sports Med* 2014;48:1294–1208.

5) Hainline B, Derman W, Vernec A, et al. International Olympic Committee Consensus Statement on pain management in elite athletes. *Br J Sports Med* 2017;51:1245–1258.

PART III

Medical and Societal Considerations of Concussion

26 Hiding Concussion (I don't want to let my teammates down)

A 22-year-old water polo player received a sharp blow to the head during a competition. This occurred during a skirmish and went unnoticed by key stakeholders on the sideline. The athlete felt disoriented, had severe headache, and was nauseated. However, he continued to play because he did not want to let his teammates down. Further, he felt that he should "tough it out" rather than give in to his symptoms. Although he completed the competition uneventfully and returned home that day, he developed increasingly severe symptoms of memory difficulty, headache, and a sense of disequilibrium. He finally sought a formal evaluation four days later.

What do you do now?

HIDING CONCUSSION

The culture of concussion safety is undergoing a paradigm shift. Decades ago, it was common knowledge that if you "had your bell rung," you simply needed to tough it out. Although some return-to-play concussion protocols were created in the 1980s and 1990s, they all provided a provision for athletes who experienced a concussion to return to play the same day. Further, it was often commonly accepted that concussion was not a serious brain injury.

This paradigm has shifted considerably in the past 10 years. All 50 states in the United States have concussion laws that mandate no return to play for an individual who has had a concussion. Further, the position and consensus statements of all medical organizations provide unequivocal guidelines that individuals cannot return to play on the same day as a concussion, and that they should undergo a graduated return-to-play protocol before returning to full competition. Despite these advances, surveys reveal that athletes are unlikely to report a concussion because of any of the following reasons: (1) they do not want to let their teammates down; (2) they believe that they are invincible or can manage their symptoms without a formal evaluation; (3) they fear taking time away from sport because they may lose their spot on the team; and (4) they are unaware of all of the symptoms of concussion.

Emerging information reveals that athletes who self-report concussion immediately are able to return to play at least two days earlier than those who do not self-report immediately. Other emerging data reveal that athletes who undergo a supervised, structured return-to-play protocol return to full activities much sooner than those who undergo an unstructured recovery and return to play protocol. In other words, early concussion management and intervention allow earlier clinical recovery. This alone is compelling information to encourage athletes to self-report concussion. Although the culture of concussion safety has improved considerably, all stakeholders, including athletes, need to be educated about the dangers of not self-reporting concussion, and the benefits of doing so. Because we lack consensus on how best to improve concussion safety, the NCAA and Department of Defense have funded research and educational studies (e.g., the NCAA-DoD Mind

Matters Challenge) to provide an evidence-based approach regarding the norms and culture of concussion safety.

TAKE-HOME POINTS

· Although policies and education regarding concussion safety have improved considerably during the past decade, athletes continue to hide concussion.
· Athletes who self-report concussion return to play sooner than athletes who do not.
· Evidence-based interventions are needed to shift perceived norms and continue to improve the culture of concussion safety.

Further Reading

1) Torres DM, Galetta KM, Phillips HW, et al. Sports-related concussion: anonymous survey of a collegiate cohort. *Neur Clin Practice* 2013;3:279–287.
2) Hainline B, Dexter WW, DiFiori J. Sports-related concussion: truth be told. *Neur Clin Practice* 2013;3:277–278.
3) NCAA and DoD launch concussion study. http://www.ncaa.org/about/resources/media-center/news/ncaa-dod-launch-concussion-study. Accessed September 15, 2019.

27 Independent Medical Care (My coach keeps pushing me to get back to practice)

A 27-year-old professional female soccer player complained to her team physician that the coach was placing undue pressure on her to return to practice, even though she did not feel fit to do so. She suffered two concussions in the same season, and never recovered fully. She had ongoing symptoms of dizziness and imbalance, and felt incapable of making strategic decisions. She had been unable to advance fully in a return-to-play protocol. Neurologic evaluation was unremarkable. The coach was placing increasing pressure on the player, stating that she owes it to the coach, the team, and the sponsors to play because she is a paid professional athlete. She is quite conflicted between her sense of well-being, her sense of duty, and the pressure being placed on her by the coach.

What do you do now?

INDEPENDENT MEDICAL CARE

There is an evolving paradigm shift regarding athlete-centered medicine. Whereas coaches have often had considerable influence over the hiring and firing of medical personnel and medical decision-making, this culture is no longer viable. Independent medical care should be the guiding principle for both individual and team sports. The cornerstone of independent medical care is that the primary athletics health-care providers have unchallengeable, autonomous authority to make all medical and return-to-play decisions. Medical decisions should always be established independently of the coach and in the sole interest of the athlete, and medical lines of authority should be transparent. While it is appropriate for the coach to ask the treating clinician for a general update, the coach should not try to influence medical decision-making.

The following 10 statements are paraphrased from the *Inter-Association Consensus Statement on Best Practices for Sports Medicine Management for Secondary Schools and Colleges*. These principles can be applied at every level of sport.

1. The physical and psychosocial welfare of the individual athlete should always be the highest priority of the athletic trainer, other clinicians, and the team physician.
2. Any program that delivers athletic training services to athletes should always have a designated medical director.
3. Sports medicine physicians, athletic trainers, and other clinicians should always practice in a manner that integrates the best current research evidence within the preferences and values of each athlete.
4. The clinical responsibilities of an athletic trainer and other non-physician clinicians should always be performed in a manner that is consistent with the written or verbal instructions of a physician or standing orders and clinical management protocols that have been approved by a program's designated medical director.
5. Decisions that affect the current or future health status of an athlete who has an injury or illness should only be made by a properly credentialed health professional (e.g., a physician,

an athletic trainer, or other clinician who has a physician's authorization to make the decision).

6. In every case that a physician has granted an athletic trainer or other clinician the discretion to make decisions relating to an individual athlete's injury management or sports participation status, all aspects of the care process and changes in the athlete's disposition should be thoroughly documented.

7. Coaches must not be allowed to impose demands that are inconsistent with guidelines and recommendations established by sports medicine and athletic training professional organizations.

8. An athletic trainer's role delineation and employment status (and that of other non-physician clinicians) should be determined through a formal administrative role for a physician who provides medical direction.

9. The medical provider's professional qualifications and performance evaluations must not be primarily judged by administrative personnel who lack health-care expertise, particularly in the context of hiring, promotion, and termination decisions.

10. Schools and clubs should adopt an administrative structure for delivery of integrated sports medicine and athletic training services to minimize the potential for any conflicts of interest that could adversely affect the health and well-being of student-athletes.

TAKE-HOME POINTS

· There is an evolving cultural shift to an athlete-centered approach to sports medicine.
· Independent medical care is founded on the principle that coaches have no authority in medical decision-making.
· Primary athletics health-care providers should have unchallengeable, autonomous authority for all medical and return-to-play decisions.

Further Reading

1) Courson R et al. Inter-association consensus statement on best practices for sports medicine management for secondary schools and colleges. *J Athl Train* 2014;49:128–137.

2) Independent Medical Care Legislation. A briefing document submitted by: The Committee on Competitive Safeguards and Medical Aspects of Sports and the NCAA Sport Science Institute. http://www.ncaa.org/sites/default/files/SSI_IMC-Briefing-Document_All-Divisions%C2%AD_20170405.pdf.

28 Multiple Concussions and Retirement from Sport (My daughter has had four concussions)

The mother of a 19-year-old field hockey player accompanied her daughter for a discussion about continued sport participation. The daughter had her first concussion at age 16 and had two subsequent concussions each year thereafter. She recovered uneventfully from each. She had her fourth concussion three weeks prior to the evaluation, after a seemingly minor collision with a teammate. She immediately developed a sense of disequilibrium with a pounding headache and blurred vision. Her symptoms have persisted despite rest and an attempted gradual exercise protocol. The mother wanted guidance regarding retirement from all contact sports.

What do you do now?

MULTIPLE CONCUSSIONS AND RETIREMENT FROM SPORT

There is perhaps no more vexing or contentious aspect of concussion management than deciding about retirement from sport because of multiple concussions. Because the neurobiology of concussion remains poorly defined, and there are no objective biomarkers of short-term or long-term sequelae of concussion or repetitive concussion, no objective guidance is available. Further, there are no clear-cut consensus guidelines on this matter. Anecdotally, some people state that retirement should occur after three concussions, but others state that such a number is artificial, and lacks scientific merit.

The international Concussion in Sport Group has not weighed in on this matter. The position statement from the American Medical Society for Sports Medicine does have a section on disqualification from sport, which notes the lack of evidence-based guidelines for disqualifying or retiring an athlete from sport after concussion, and that each athlete should be individually assessed. They further state that there is no set number of concussions or repetitive head impact exposures that should force retirement.

Table 28.1 provides some emerging considerations that guide decision-making regarding retirement from sport because of concussion. Key

TABLE 28.1 **Retirement Considerations Following Multiple Concussions**

Guidance for Retirement from Sport	Guidance for Continued Sport Participation
Evidence of worrisome neurologic deficit, behavioral changes, or post-traumatic seizures	Concussion symptoms resolve in timely and satisfactory manner
Prolonged recovery following concussion	Long interval between concussions
Low threshold for developing concussion	Education regarding concussion and head-impact exposure safety
Shortened time intervals between concussions	Desire to continue playing/ competing in contact-collision sport
MRI findings of diffuse axonal injury, frontotemporal gliosis, arteriovenous malformation, or other vascular risk factors	

considerations include prolonged recovery and lowered threshold for developing a concussion. The development of objective neurological sequelae is also an important factor to consider. Finally, individual and family fears may outweigh all other considerations.

The largest and most detailed prospective longitudinal concussion study in history is being done in the NCAA–Department of Defense CARE Consortium. This study assesses NCAA student-athletes and tactical athletes from the service academies on clinical grounds, and is obtaining detailed objective biomarkers (e.g., genetics, genomics, blood biomarkers, brain MRI, and head accelerometry) from those in high-risk sports. Athletes in high-risk sports who suffer a concussion will be compared to athletes in the same sports who have never had a concussion, and athletes in low-risk sports (e.g., tennis) who have not suffered a concussion and lack repetitive head-impact exposure. It is through such studies that we can begin to form evidence-informed decisions about retirement from sport due to concussion. In the interim, we need to balance caution, safety, and avoidance of fear-based decisions.

Further Reading

1) Harmon KG, Clugston JR, Dec K, et al. American Medical Society for Sports Medicine position statement on concussion in sport. *Br J Sports Med* 2019;53:213–225.

2) Davis-Hayes C, Baker DR, Bottiglieri TS, et al. Medical retirement from sport after concussions: a practical guide for a difficult discussion. *Neurol Clin Pract* 2018;8:40–47.

3) Cantu RC, Register-Mihalik JK. Considerations for return-to-play and retirement decisions after concussion. *PM&R* 2011;3:S440–S444.

4) Broglio SP, McCrea M, McAllister T, Harezlak J, Katz B, Hack D, Hainline B. A national study on the effects of concussion in collegiate athletes and US military service academy members: the NCAA-DoD Concussion Assessment, Research and Education (CARE) Consortium structure and methods. *Sports Med* 2017;47:1437–1451.

29 Repetitive Head Impact Exposure (Should I be worried that my son's football play may cause long-term brain damage?)

A father asked to consult with a primary care sports medicine physician regarding his 18-year-old son. The son was scheduled to begin playing college football, but the father had several concerns. The son denied ever having suffered a concussion, and he excelled academically. The father said that he was not concerned about concussion, but rather about repetitive head impact exposure. He cited statistics that high school football athletes are exposed to about 600 repetitive head impacts per season. The father is convinced that such exposure will lead to long-term brain damage, and he wanted the sports medicine physician's input.

What do you do now?

REPETITIVE HEAD IMPACT EXPOSURE

We do not understand the natural history of concussion, nor the neurobiology of concussion. When we return an athlete to play, we do so with good confidence that the athlete has recovered clinically, but we do not know if the athlete has recovered neurobiologically because we have no objective biomarkers of concussion. The same is true for repetitive head impact exposure.

Repetitive head impact exposure refers to head impacts that are greater than 15 g (1 g is the force of gravity). Sometimes called subconcussive trauma, such impact causes no visible signs or symptoms of concussion but may hypothetically damage the brain's structural integrity. We do not have an ideal way of measuring both linear and rotational acceleration that occurs with head impact exposure. The Head Impact Telemetry System (HITS) has been studied more than any other system for this purpose, but the measurements are indirect. The HITS system depends on head accelerometers placed in a football helmet, and thus may measure helmet movement rather than skull and brain movement. Other devices, including accelerometers placed in the mastoid region, or as mouth guards, have not yet provided meaningful data.

Retrospective studies have tried to estimate the amount of head impact exposure an athlete may have undergone, and to correlate such estimates with a post-mortem or ante-mortem disease state, but this is an imprecise exercise. In short-term prospective studies, repetitive head impact exposure without clinical concussion can lead to within-season alterations in brain activation during performance of a visual working memory task, in a functional magnetic resonance imaging (MRI) exam. Similarly, changes in white matter integrity have been observed in athletes exposed to repetitive head impact without clinical concussion. It remains unclear if such neuroimaging changes remain stable, return to baseline, or worsen over time.

The NCAA–DoD CARE Consortium is the only prospective, longitudinal concussion study to compare the effects of concussion and repetitive head impact exposure without concussion, and the effects of training at an elite level without either concussion or repetitive head impact exposure. This landmark study is gathering data on the quantity of head impact exposure while measuring serial brain MRI studies (both quantitative and qualitative), blood biomarkers, detailed clinical data, and genetic and genomic characteristics.

We have no consensus about the risk of repetitive head impact exposure, nor are there concrete guidelines about this matter. The position statement of the American Medical Society for Sports Medicine states that the short-term and long-term effects of repetitive head impacts cannot be accurately characterized using current technology, and that future research is needed. The international consensus from the Concussion in Sport Group states that there is much more to learn about the potential causes and effects of repetitive head impact exposure.

Although we have no concrete answers, and there are no evidence- or consensus-based guidelines on this matter, it is prudent to mitigate head impact exposure. Such mitigation centers around a "safety first" approach to practice and competition. There should be no gratuitous contact in practice, and there is no place in sport for deliberately inflicting injury on the opponent. As much as possible, the head needs to be taken out of the game of football and other contact/collision sports. Coaches and other stakeholders need to be educated about possible short-term and long-term sequelae of repetitive head impact exposure. Ultimately, parents and athletes need to make decisions based on their assessment of the current knowledge, and they can be further guided by the willingness and passion of the athlete to compete, coupled with the culture of safety in the athlete's team.

TAKE-HOME POINTS

· Repetitive head impact exposure refers to the transfer of mechanical energy to the brain without clinical concussion, with possible axonal or neuronal injury.
· Short-term brain changes on MRI exams have been identified in athletes with a history of repetitive head impact exposure, but it is not clear if these changes normalize, stay static, or worsen over time.
· There is no known causal correlation between repetitive head impact exposure and long-term neurological disease.
· A "safety first" approach should always be taken in sport, and decisions to play should be guided by the individual's willingness and passion to play, coupled with the team's culture of safety.

Further Reading

1) Nauman EA, Talavage TM. Subconcussive trauma. In Hainline B, Stern RA (Eds.), *Sports Neurology*, San Diego: Elsevier BV, 2018, pp 245–255.

2) Harmon KG, Clugston JR, Dec K, et al. American Medical Society for Sports Medicine position statement on concussion in sport. *Br J Sports Med* 2019;53:213–225.

3) McCrory P, Meeuwisse W, Dvorak J, et al. Consensus statement on concussion in sport—the 5th international conference on concussion in sport held in Berlin, October 2016.

30 Protective Equipment (Shouldn't my son get a new football helmet?)

During a pre-participation physical examination, the father asked the pediatrician to write a letter on behalf of his 15-year-old son and the son's team to the football coach. The father had recently read about new football helmet standards developed by the National Football League (NFL). He noted that the helmets used by his son's team were in the "red" category of the NFL guidance (meaning no longer recommended). He felt that a letter from the pediatrician would help convince the coach that the highest-rated NFL helmets should be used for his son's football team.

What you do now?

PROTECTIVE EQUIPMENT

In the 1930s, there was considerable debate regarding the introduction of a rigid plastic helmet into American football. Some believed that such a helmet was necessary to prevent brain injury, and others cautioned that it could be used as a weapon. Ultimately, the NCAA and the NFL adopted a rigid plastic helmet as mandatory equipment, and this has become the standard for all levels of the game.

There is no question that football helmets—and helmets used in other sports such as skiing/snowboarding, cycling, motor racing, and ice hockey—mitigate catastrophic brain injury. Helmet safety standards have been developed to prevent focal head injury from high linear forces, thereby protecting against skull fractures and intracerebral hematomas. However, helmets have not been designed to prevent concussion.

There is emerging information that the use of helmets in sport may have shifted athletes' risk from catastrophic injury to concussion and repetitive head impact exposure. Risk-taking behavior changes with protective equipment, and this includes using the head as a weapon when a helmet is worn. Further, protocols for testing helmet safety were established with linear head acceleration-based metrics. Helmets are not designed to protect against low-energy collisions; thus, they may provide inadequate protection in common player-to-player collisions. Further, helmets do not protect against rotational injuries; these injuries may be most responsible for axonal damage and long-term neurobehavioral outcomes of traumatic brain injury.

The National Operating Committee on Standards for Athletic Equipment (NOCSAE) is an independent and nonprofit standards-development body that seeks to enhance athletic safety through scientific research and the creation of performance standards for athletic equipment. It is standard practice for contact/collision sports to mandate that protective helmets are certified by NOCSAE. Whereas the NOCSAE standard has historically focused on linear acceleration, very recently they have introduced rotational acceleration thresholds into their certification standards for new football helmets. The NFL also has developed standards independent of NOCSAE, and they provide recommendations (but not certification) for football helmets worn by NFL players. However, the NFL recommendations are based on the expected physics of a professional football player, and it is not clear that their data are relevant to youth, high school, or even collegiate football.

What is important to understand is that helmets prevent catastrophic brain injury, but at present have a marginal impact on mitigating concussion risk. Helmets are updated and certified annually—a necessary but insufficient step in creating safe play in contact/collision sports. Ultimately, the head needs to be taken out of the game.

TAKE-HOME POINTS

· Helmets are designed to mitigate skull fractures and catastrophic brain injury.
· Helmets are not designed to protect against concussion.
· Helmets are sometimes used as a weapon.
· To mitigate concussion risk in contact/collision sports, the head needs to be taken out of the game.

Further Reading
1) Karton C, Hoshizaki TB. Concussive and subconcussive brain trauma: the complexity of impact biomechanics and injury risk in contact sport. In Hainline B, Stern RA (Eds.), *Sports Neurology*, San Diego: Elsevier EV, 2018, pp 39–49.
2) National Operating Committee on Standards for Athletic Equipment (NOCSAE). Football helmets standards overview. https://nocsae.org/wp-content/uploads/2018/05/NOCSAE-Summary-of-Procedures-for-Adoption-and-Implementation-of-Standard.pdf.

31 Youth Tackle Football (Can you please sign this petition to ban youth tackle football?)

During a routine office visit, the mother of a 10-year-old boy asked a pediatrician to sign a petition to ban youth tackle football. She expressed concern that youth tackle football is associated with brain degeneration later in life. She cited an influential media outlet that described a long-term study indicating such results. She expressed the view that there is no moral justification for exposing our youth to certain long-term brain problems. She sought not to discuss the issues with the pediatrician, just to obtain a signature on the petition.

What do you do now?

YOUTH TACKLE FOOTBALL

Each year in the United States, 44 million youth participate in sports. Youth sports provide a foundation for physical literacy, defined as the motivation, confidence, physical competence, knowledge, and understanding to value and take responsibility for engagement in lifelong physical activity. Physical literacy is highly associated with a later decreased likelihood of drug use, school dropout, poor work performance, and chronic medical conditions, especially metabolic syndrome. It is noteworthy that currently, approximately 50% of individuals who wish to serve in the US Armed Forces cannot do so because of physical illiteracy.

Although physical literacy is not tied to sport alone, there are limited opportunities to develop physical literacy in the United States since physical education classes at school have been limited. Currently, only 25% of high school students meet the minimum recommendations for exercise. Thus, full participation in youth sport appears to be a natural antidote to the profound negative long-term effects of physical illiteracy.

That being said, the safety of youth sports must be a prime consideration. There is growing concern about this subject, especially with regard to catastrophic injury, including traumatic brain injury. The culture of safety must be paramount, especially in youth sports, and should be deeply ingrained within all key stakeholders, especially coaches and officials.

Football is one of the most popular sports in the United States, with 5 million youth playing annually. Although it provides an important foundation for developing physical literacy and long-term participation in sport, it is also associated with inherent risk, especially during the act of tackling or being tackled. Tackling is associated with an overall increased risk of musculoskeletal injuries and head and neck injuries. Although it is assumed that tackling in youth football is associated with an increased risk of repetitive head impact exposure, this assumption has not been validated at the youth level.

In 2017, a survey study compared individuals who had played American football before or after the age of 12, and revealed increased odds of clinically meaningful impairments in behavioral regulation, apathy, executive function, and depression in those who began playing at a younger age.

Prominent media coverage linked these results to findings in an autopsy study of former professional football players, in which 110 of 111 brains had neuropathologic evidence findings of chronic traumatic encephalopathy. What has received little media coverage is the policy statement from the Council on Sports Medicine and Fitness within the American Academy of Pediatrics. This 2015 policy statement was based on a careful analysis of the risks versus benefits of youth tackle football. Ultimately, the policy statement did not recommend removing tackling from youth football, but rather recommended a multipronged approach to improving the safety of youth football.

Whereas the elimination of youth tackle football would have previously seemed either unthinkable or not a priority, more recent evidence indicates that most parents believe that youth tackle football should be banned. Yet to date, the science regarding possible causal effects of long-term brain or behavioral effects of youth tackle football has been flawed. Sample selection has been biased, no control groups were included, and there has been no consideration of other risk factors of long-term brain and behavioral dysfunction. Even the authors of the 2017 study state that their results "should not be used to inform safety or policy decision in regards to youth football."

At present, it is desirable to develop a consensus based on existing scientific evidence. One well-designed model is the American Development Model (see Appendix 31.1), which is based on the concept of long-term athlete development. Long-term athlete development has become a more universally accepted goal in youth-level sport. Its basic principles are that early exposure to youth sport should be fun, and focused on developing athleticism (i.e., agility, balance, coordination, speed, stamina, and strength) rather than mastery of a single sport.

USA Hockey was the first national governing body to apply the principles of long-term athlete development to an American sport. In essence, the American Development Model for youth hockey stated that youth hockey should not be played like adult hockey. As a result, USA Hockey developed several novel strategies, such as changing the length of the ice rink to the current width of adult hockey and limiting the amount of exposure to hockey play in general, especially hockey contact. Other sports such as tennis, golf, basketball, baseball, and swimming have increasingly adopted this model.

The American Development Model incorporates the following concepts:

- Universal access to create opportunity for athletes
- Developmentally appropriate activities that emphasize motor and foundational skills
- Multisport or multi-activity participation that is cross-training
- Fun, engaging, and progressively challenging atmosphere
- High-quality coaching at all age levels.

Currently, the Football Development Model Council, under the umbrella of USA Football, is systematically addressing the state of knowledge about tackling and youth football. One of the authors (BH) is chair. This Council includes prominent neuroscientists and youth sport stakeholders and well-known college football coaches who have eliminated tackling during football practice. The Council's goal is to understand how to purposefully and incrementally teach athletes to engage in contact in football, in a manner that is both developmentally appropriate and safe. Fundamentally, many sports involve contact and collision, including ice hockey, lacrosse, soccer, football, and wrestling. Thus, the purpose is not to eliminate all contact/collision sports, but rather to use science and policy to improve safety while allowing engagement in activities that have a positive long-term impact on health.

TAKE-HOME POINTS

- Physical illiteracy is a health, economic, and national defense threat.
- Youth sport can improve physical literacy, and should be conducted in a manner that emphasizes safety.
- The scientific consensus around youth tackle football has been overshadowed by inaccurate media reports.
- The American Development Model provides a sound framework for developing policies and procedures for all youth sport, including football.

APPENDIX 31.1: THE AMERICAN DEVELOPMENT MODEL

Reprinted with permission, Coaching Education, United States Olympic Committee

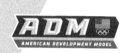

REBUILDING ATHLETES IN AMERICA

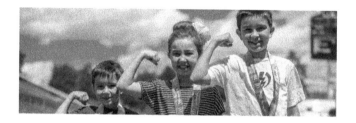

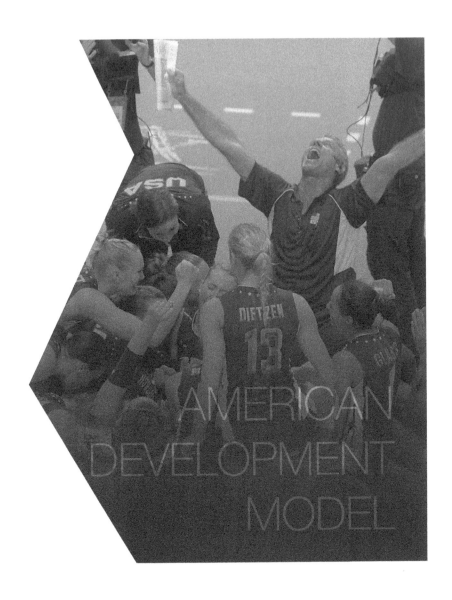

AMERICAN
DEVELOPMENT
MODEL

TABLE OF CONTENTS

STATE OF THE GAMES: WHY CREATE ADM?

The American Development Model is a concerted effort between the United States Olympic Committee and its National Governing Bodies of sport to apply long-term athlete development principles in a way that resonates with the culture of sport in the United States.

The ADM is influenced by the work of Istvan Balyi, who is known worldwide as an industry leader in long-term athlete development principles. Balyi's approach to organized sport focuses on key principles of development and periodization of training plans, which help support athletes' individual needs.

The need to rethink how we organize, operate and execute sport activity in the United States has been a point of emphasis over the last 15 years. The call to action became more urgent in 2013, when the Aspen Project Play Initiative hosted a gathering of sports organizations and administrators to discuss key issues facing sport in the U.S. The following conclusions from that meeting were the inspiration behind the ADM:

FROM PROJECT PLAY REPORT: 2015 (www.aspenprojectplay.org)

Falling Sport Participation Rates
Some of the most widely practiced sports in the U.S. were seeing major declines in participation due to organized sport programs centered around the most talented, well-resourced athletes.

Decline in Participation Rates Among Children ages 6-12 between 2008-2013

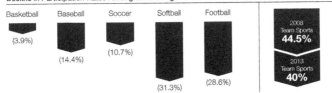

Basketball	Baseball	Soccer	Softball	Football
(3.9%)	(14.4%)	(10.7%)	(31.3%)	(28.6%)

2008 Team Sports **44.5%**

2013 Team Sports **40%**

According to Sports & Fitness Industry Association (SFIA), children ages 6 to 12 who played team sports regularly fell from 44.5 percent in 2008 to 40 percent in 2013.

Obesity Crisis

Childhood obesity rates nearly tripled. The percentage of obese children ages 6-11 increased from 7 percent in 1980 to 18 percent in 2010. Among children ages 12 to 19, that figure grew from 5 percent to 18 percent (*Centers for Disease Control and Prevention, 2015*). One study found that among 17 developed nations, **the U.S. had the highest rates of childhood obesity among those ages 5-19** (*National Academy of Sciences, 2013*).

Low Physical Activity Rates

Starting at age 9 — when children often develop a self-concept of whether or not they are an athlete — physical activity rates begin to drop sharply. By age 15, moderate-to-vigorous physical activity declines 75 percent, a higher rate than in Europe (*Designed to Move, 2012*). At that point, they average only 49 minutes per weekday and 35 minutes per weekend (*Journal of the American Medical Association, 2008*). Among kids ages 6-17, one in five youth are considered inactive, meaning they report no physical activity (*Physical Activity Council, 2015*). Further, only one in three children is physically active every day (*Fitness.gov*). Among high school students, that figure drops to nearly 29 percent. Meanwhile, more children each year are completely inactive, with one in five youth ages 6-17 not engaging in any activity, according to SFIA. In 2014, the number of inactives ages 6+ grew to 28.3 percent (82.7 million) of the U.S. population — the highest rate in the last six years (*Physical Activity Council, 2015*).

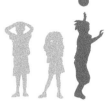

Shorter Lives

Today's children could be the **first generation to live shorter, less healthy lives than their parents** due to obesity and other related diseases. (*Designed to Move, 2012*)

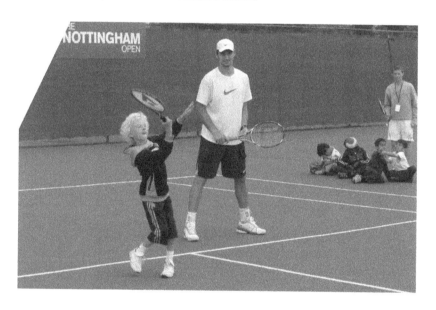

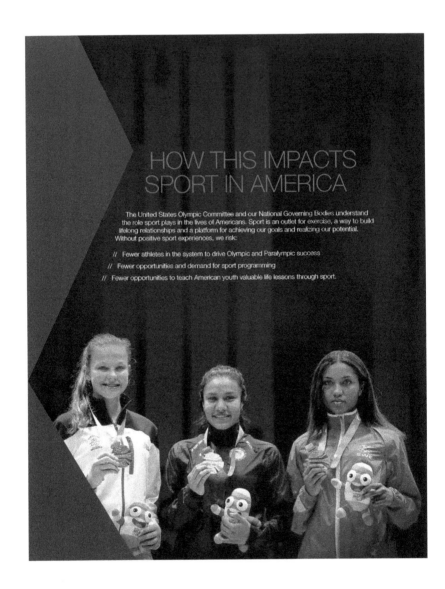

HOW THIS IMPACTS
SPORT IN AMERICA

The United States Olympic Committee and our National Governing Bodies understand the role sport plays in the lives of Americans. Sport is an outlet for exercise, a way to build lifelong relationships and a platform for achieving our goals and realizing our potential. Without positive sport experiences, we risk:

// Fewer athletes in the system to drive Olympic and Paralympic success

// Fewer opportunities and demand for sport programming

// Fewer opportunities to teach American youth valuable life lessons through sport.

OVERVIEW

The United States Olympic Committee, in partnership with the National Governing Bodies, created the American Development Model in 2014 to help Americans realize their full athletic potential and utilize sport as a path toward an active and healthy lifestyle.

The model utilizes long-term athlete development concepts to promote sustained physical activity, participation in sport, and Olympic and Paralympic success. These concepts have been tailored to create a framework for developing American youth through sport.

The American Development Model is comprised of four key elements:

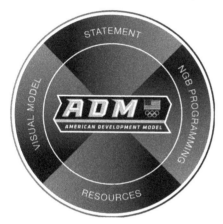

The ultimate goal is to create positive experiences for American athletes at every level. By using the American Development Model, clubs, coaches and parents can help maximize potential for future elite athletes, and improve the health and well-being for future generations in the United States.

The purpose of this document is to provide key influencers – including administrators, coaches and parents – a roadmap for building and delivering programs that focus on the individual athlete at each stage of development. The physical, emotional and mental landscape of each stage should enhance the athlete's overall development, while creating positive experiences in sport.

ADM STATEMENT

The United States Olympic Committee and its National Governing Bodies embrace the athlete development principles that allow American youth to utilize sport as a path toward an active and healthy lifestyle, and create opportunities for athletes to maximize their full potential. These five key principles include:

// Universal access to create opportunity for all athletes

// Developmentally appropriate activities that emphasize motor and foundational skills

// Multi-sport or multi-activity participation (i.e. cross-training)

// Fun, engaging and progressively challenging atmosphere

// Quality coaching at all age levels

By creating early positive experiences for all athletes, the American Development Model will keep more children engaged in sport longer with four outcomes:

// Grow both the general athlete population and the pool of elite athletes from which future U.S. Olympians and Paralympians are selected

// Develop fundamental skills that transfer between sports

// Provide an appropriate avenue to fulfill an individual's athletic potential

// Create a generation that loves sport and physical activity, and transfers that passion to the next generation

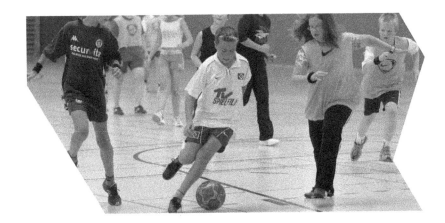

KEY PRINCIPLES

I.   UNIVERSAL ACCESS TO CREATE OPPORTUNITY FOR ALL ATHLETES

Universal access is defined as creating opportunities for everyone to participate in sport. By providing universal access to all youth regardless of gender, race, physical disability, and economic status, more children could become involved in sport and be more physically active. Sport must be inclusive so that all children have the opportunity to discover the benefit of physical activity and realize their full athletic potential. Sport and physical activity are tools for children to express themselves, develop social relationships and learn valuable life lessons.

II.   DEVELOPMENTALLY APPROPRIATE ACTIVITIES THAT EMPHASIZE MOTOR AND FOUNDATIONAL SKILL DEVELOPMENT

A clear understanding of an individual's developmental level (as opposed to his or her age) will help coaches, parents and administrators appropriately tailor the training, skills and tactics taught to maximize an individual's full potential, while helping avoid burnout.

In order to succeed, athletes must first learn foundational motor skills and technique. Coaches, parents and administrators who jump directly into competition tactics and strategy without emphasizing basic fundamentals may put their child or athlete at a disadvantage. To ensure long-term success, athletes must be given adequate time and knowledge to develop these essential building blocks for success.

III.   ENCOURAGE MULTI-SPORT PARTICIPATION

Multi-sport participation is critical to developing a well-rounded foundation for physical activity that can transfer between sports. Encouraging children to participate in multiple sport activities at a young age offers them the opportunity to explore, play and discover sport according to their personal interests and skill level.

Multi-sport play also provides several cross-training benefits for athletes – such as strength, endurance, agility, coordination and speed training — that enhances athleticism and promotes a healthy lifestyle. Athletes also benefit from the social and psychological impact of multi-sport participation.

IV.   FUN, ENGAGING AND CHALLENGING ATMOSPHERE

A fun, engaging and challenging environment is essential for any youth sport activity. The definition of "fun" may change as children advance to more elite levels of competition, but a standard emphasis on making the process positive and enjoyable is key.

Free and spontaneous play is encouraged to help foster growth and development. By offering the opportunity for unstructured play, athletes are more likely to customize physical activity to meet their needs and keep the "fun" in sport intact. Creating a team mentality through positive reinforcement is also critical.

Consult your sport's National Governing Body for suggestions on age-appropriate dose and duration of practice and competition to help avoid burnout.

V.   QUALITY COACHING AT ALL AGE LEVELS

Quality coaches are critical to athlete development; therefore quality coaching education is critical for athlete success at all competitive levels. Quality coaching not only requires a youth coach to be qualified and highly knowledgeable of their sport, but also basic training on effective communication, practice planning and athlete development. The very best coaches view themselves as continual learners and are always working toward improving themselves. Consult your sport's National Governing Body for information on the different types of coaching education that are offered and/or required for your sport.

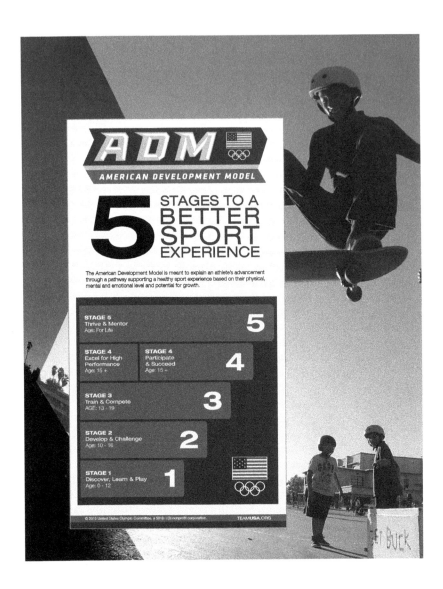

WHAT DO I DO NOW? **CONCUSSION**

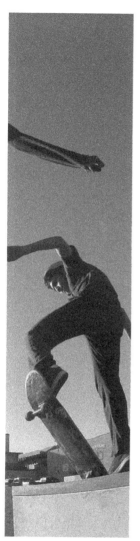

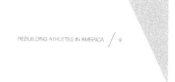

STAGES

The ADM is comprised of five stages designed to create a healthy sport experience and support an athlete's advancement based on their physical, mental and emotional level, and potential for growth.

Pathway models like the ADM 5 Stages should be used to reference what key concepts athletes should be focused, encouraged or organized around as they develop and grow in their sports experiences. The pathway models are guides to explain how athletes navigate development and competitive expectations as they journey in the sport.

Consumers can use pathway models to understand at what developmental stages an athlete should consider focusing on skill development vs. competition, or at what ages one could expect to become more focused on elite performance.

Every sport will have a different pathway for development and navigation will be different for each sport experience, and this is ok. The ADM 5 stage model is a guideline for sports in America to use to encourage development and pathway guidance.

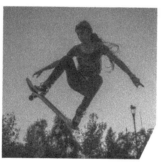

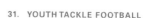

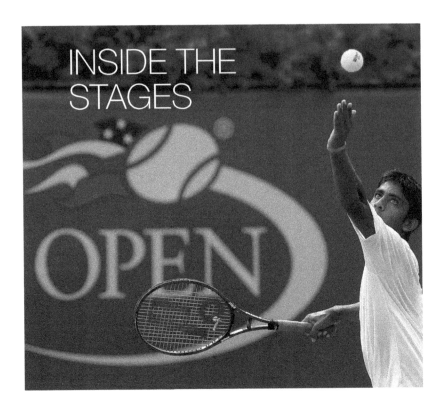

STAGE 1: DISCOVER, LEARN AND PLAY (AGES 0-12)

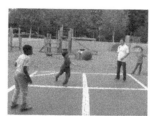

This is the first step to being involved with sports at a young age (0-12) or when first introduced to a new sport. Discovery of key concepts and motor skills of the sport/activity is critical in order to learn how the sport is played. Many skills are transferrable between sports. Programs should accommodate athletes that participate in multiple sports. This early stage requires coaching that will allow fun and enjoyment through discovery and exploration.

ATHLETE
// Learning basic rules and sport techniques
// Play multiple sports to accelerate motor skill development
// Emphasize skill development, sport education and age-appropriate play
// Emphasize practice over competition; if competing, not beyond local or regional levels
// Encourage deliberate play

DISCOVER
// Have fun
// Sample multiple sports through unstructured play
// Develop motor skills that transfer from sport to sport
// Cultivate a passion for sport and an active lifestyle
// Socialize with others
// Utilize free or spontaneous play for discovery of the sport and new skills

LEARN
// Core fundamental movements
// How to use size and age-appropriate equipment, and playing surfaces
// Rules of the game

PLAY
// Physical education class
// Open gym
// Free/spontaneous play
// Basic organized play
// Everyone has an equal chance to play in competition

STAGE 2: DEVELOP AND CHALLENGE (AGES 10-16)

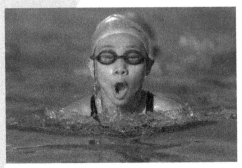 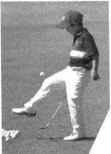

The second stage of the development process occurs after an athlete has been engaged in a sport and wants to explore more organized training options. This stage focuses on refining the skills needed to be successful in the activity or sport, and then furthering skill development through challenges, such as recreational competition, organized sport programs or club participation.

Athlete readiness and motivation determine the choice to pursue the next level in sport. The second stage may begin earlier for some athletes who are quick to develop physically and mentally. Fun and socialization are still key areas of emphasis in order to encourage future participation and avoid burnout.

ATHLETE
// Understand rules and techniques of the sport
// Participate in multiple sports for continued motor and physical development
// Participate in a fun, structured and ongoing training program (as opposed to participating in open gym)
// Compete at local and regional levels
// Emphasize practice and skill development over competing
// Understand the impact on performance due to different maturation rates

DEVELOP
// Physical: Core movement fundamentals, increasing requirements for speed, agility, balance, endurance, strength and coordination
// Psychological and social: interpersonal skills, teamwork, communication skills and adapting to the growing challenges of sport development
// Technical skills: Identify personal strengths and areas to improve with a continued emphasis on proper movement mechanics
// Tactical: Institute age-appropriate times for practice and competition to enhance both team and individual skill development.

CHALLENGE
// Recreational competition at local and regional levels
// Organized league play

Note: Seek challenging competition that is commensurate with the athlete and/or team.

STAGE 3: TRAIN AND COMPETE (AGES 13-19)

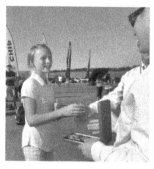 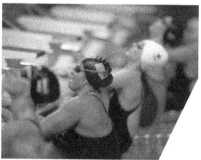

At stage three, athletes begin to train and compete in a program that matches their personal interests, goals and developmental needs. Competitions become more clearly defined in this process with potential for new experiences in team selection. Maximizing potential becomes an option for athletes as they start to grasp the commitment necessary for certain sports, and the skill sets needed to excel at the next competitive level. Technical, tactical, physical and psycho-social development becomes increasingly more important for the athlete at this time. This is also the stage to increase sport-specific training. Recreation and multi-sport play can continue to be used in a cross-training capacity to allow athletes the opportunity to more fully develop.

ATHLETE
// Begin to focus on particular sports
// Use multiple-sport play for cross-sport development
// Participate in a fun, structured and continuous training program
// Compete in more challenging situations
// Improve skills at the local, regional and/or national levels

TRAIN
// Seek opportunities to further develop skills
// Focused training through coaching
// Follow a consistent training schedule
// Increase sport-specific training
// Emphasize competition skills
// Utilize more sport-science related information such as nutrition and sport psychology
// Participate in development camps

COMPETE
// Club competition
// Middle and high school competitions
// Local, regional and national competitions

Note: Seek challenging competition that is commensurate with the athlete and or team's skills.

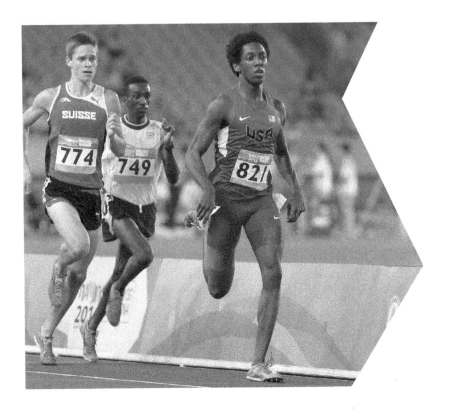

STAGE 4: EXCEL FOR HIGH PERFORMANCE OR PARTICIPATE AND SUCCEED (AGES 15+)

When an athlete reaches high school they will likely face the option to either focus on sport for high performance and increased competition, or continue to compete for the fun, healthy and social aspects of sport. Athletes will be able to choose the pathway that best represents their interests and abilities. Growth spurts, experience or dedication to training may all affect which path an athlete follows during their sport career. This stage allows for both full development and commitment to their sport(s), and enjoyment of the benefits that sport offers. Fun and socialization remain key elements of this stage, although the definition of fun changes from athlete to athlete and also will adjust based on the commitment level to high performance or participation.

EXCEL FOR HIGH PERFORMANCE

ATHLETE
// Dedicated to maximizing athletic potential
// Commit to an ongoing annual and/or long-term training program
// Is single sport-focused while in season

EXCEL
// Maximize talents
// Year-round plan to excel and progress
// Master and/or elite-level coaching
// High performance focus

HIGH PERFORMANCE
// Competitions commensurate with an athlete's skill level, and to appropriate levels outside their comfort zone
// Elite national and international competitions

PARTICIPATE AND SUCCEED

ATHLETE
// Dedicated to participating in sports to be successful and have fun
// Multiple-sport for cross-sport development
// Participate in a structured, ongoing training program
// Focus on the enjoyment of sport and the healthy benefits of participation

PARTICIPATE
// Be active and involved
// Compete for both the challenge and for fun
// Develop for personal achievement

SUCCEED
// Local- and regional-based competitions that meet the athlete's needs and their competition goals
// Sport club competition

STAGE 5: THRIVE AND MENTOR (ACTIVE FOR LIFE)

Everyone can use sport and physical activity to establish and maintain a healthy lifestyle.

Many athletes want to give back to their sport after they finish competing. Coaching, officiating and mentoring other athletes are natural next steps. With previous experience as an athlete, the coach, official and/or administrator can help prepare other athletes to be the best they can be in sport and enjoy the development process.

ATHLETE
// Transition from participant to sport leader as a coach or advocate
// Pursue opportunities to remain involved in sport
// Maintain a physically active and healthy lifestyle

MENTOR
// Certified coach
// Sport club management
// NGB involvement
// Official
// Professional development in chosen sport(s)

THRIVE
// Masters programs/competitions
// Consistent exercise
// Recreational competitions
// Personal health
// Support local and national sports and organizations

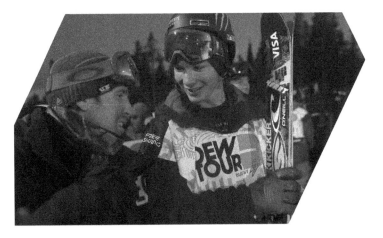

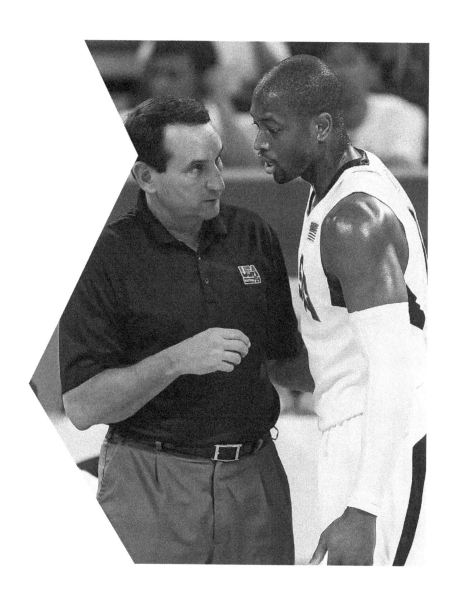

ADM AND YOU: RECOMMENDATIONS FOR IMPLEMENTATION

The United States Olympic Committee is engaging with its National Governing Bodies of sport, and sport clubs, coaches, parents and athletes in the U.S. to utilize the American Development Model in a manner that helps keep American athletes strong and inspired to achieve their personal best on and off the field of play. Use the following recommendations as a way to further your ADM advocacy in the U.S.

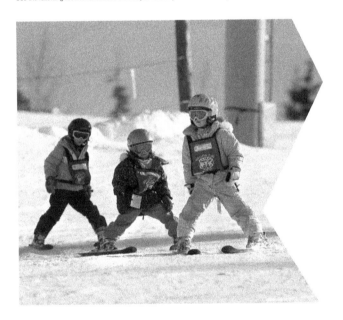

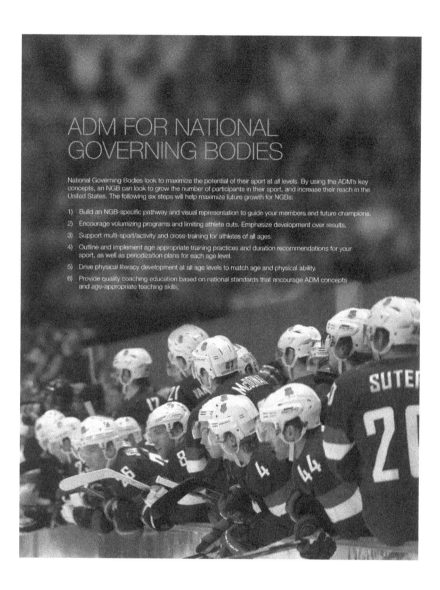

ADM FOR NATIONAL GOVERNING BODIES

National Governing Bodies look to maximize the potential of their sport at all levels. By using the ADM's key concepts, an NGB can look to grow the number of participants in their sport, and increase their reach in the United States. The following six steps will help maximize future growth for NGBs:

1) Build an NGB-specific pathway and visual representation to guide your members and future champions.

2) Encourage volumizing programs and limiting athlete cuts. Emphasize development over results.

3) Support multi-sport/activity and cross-training for athletes of all ages.

4) Outline and implement age appropriate training practices and duration recommendations for your sport, as well as periodization plans for each age level.

5) Drive physical literacy development at all age levels to match age and physical ability.

6) Provide quality coaching education based on national standards that encourage ADM concepts and age-appropriate teaching skills.

ADM FOR SPORT CLUBS

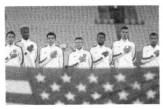

Sport clubs and organizations are a key part of both the youth and adult sport experience in the United States. By using key ADM concepts, a sport club can focus on growing their athletes and teams into success stories. Use these 10 key recommendations to help maximize your sport clubs' impact on the athlete's sport experience:

1) Limit cuts for ages 0-12 in sport programs and focus on developing skills over competition outcomes.

2) Use your NGBs sport pathway to design your own club development pathway for participation and competition offerings.

3) Provide physical literacy (i.e. agility, balance, coordination training) at every practice at every level.

4) Periodize training and rest time for your athletes to cut down on overuse injuries and burnout.

5) Encourage multi-sport/activity and cross-training to keep your athletes active and developing outside of your program.

6) Use developmentally appropriate drills and practice plans at all levels.

7) Provide qualified and certified coaches at all age levels.

8) Keep participation/competition costs reasonable. Find ways to increase numbers and retention rates from year to year, season to season.

9) Provide quality feedback and age-appropriate development benchmarks to parents and athletes.

10) Operate with an athlete-focused philosophy by creating fun, engaging and challenging sport experiences across all levels of development.

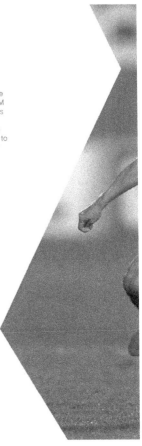

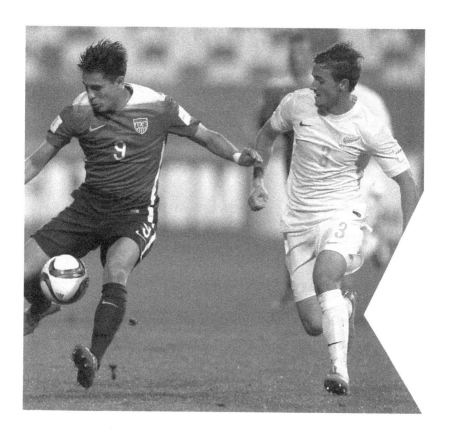

ADM FOR COACHES

Coaches hold a strong power of authority in sports. The coach's role is to maximize the potential of their athletes, while helping the athlete or team achieve the best results possible. This power of authority can make or break an athlete's sport experience. Quality coaches need to constantly develop their tools to help athletes grow and develop. The following recommendations can be used to achieve greater success in coaching:

1) Periodize training and rest time for athletes to cut down on overuse injuries and burnout.

2) Provide physical literacy (i.e. agility, balance, coordination training) at every practice at every level.

3) Use developmentally appropriate drills and practice plans at all levels.

4) Operate with an athlete-focused philosophy by creating fun, engaging and challenging sport experiences across all levels of development.

5) Provide quality feedback and age-appropriate development benchmarks to parents and athletes.

6) Focus on effort and development over outcomes to reinforce physical, technical and tactical advancements over winning.

7) Maximize athlete potential and retention at all stages of development.

8) Obtain certification as a coach and continue to develop your coaching skills, including age-appropriate teaching skills.

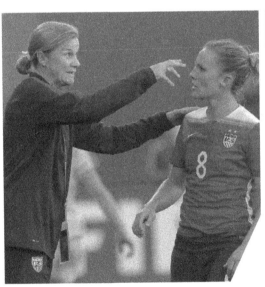
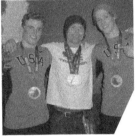

ADM FOR PARENTS

The parent's role in the sport experience can be one of support and guidance for the athlete's benefit. The following are recommendations for parents to help ensure positive sport experiences for their children:

1) Understand your child's sport pathway and recognize where they stand in terms of age and development.

2) Encourage sport sampling, in which your child plays several different sports up to age 12, at minimum, to help enhance physical literacy and to be sure they find sports they enjoy.

3) Encourage multi-sport/activity and cross-training to keep your child from burning out or developing overuse injuries.

4) Reward your child for sport development and proficiency over performance outcomes and winning.

5) Enroll your child in age-appropriate activities to ensure healthy progression and skill development before advancing to a heavy volume of competition.

6) Monitor the dose and duration your child is playing each week and encourage rest and recovery.

7) Ask for feedback from coaches and administrators on your child's development and maintain interest in your child's experience over performance outcomes.

8) Support and encourage your child to have fun. Don't forget it's about them.

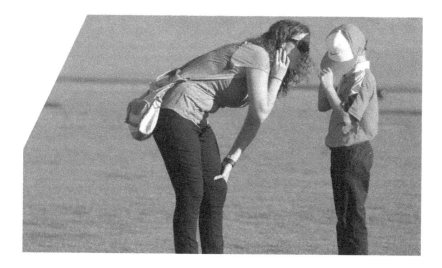

ADM FOR ATHLETES

The athlete plays the most important part in their sport experience and athletic development. At the end of the day, it is the athlete that must learn, develop and achieve physical, mental and emotional success in their sport. The following six recommendations are designed to help athletes achieve their goals and maximize their full potential in sport.

1) Develop your physical literacy and sport skills every day. Use multi-sport/activity and cross-training to help develop and achieve all-around success.

2) Focus on your skill proficiency and game development over competition results and performance outcomes at the early stages of sport development.

3) Use free-play/pick-up game opportunities to stay active and build creativity outside of structured play.

4) Listen to your body and understand that rest and recovery are part of the sport development process.

5) Set goals and gather feedback from coaches and administrators to help achieve those goals.

6) Stay active year-round and use sport as an outlet for physical activity and exercise.

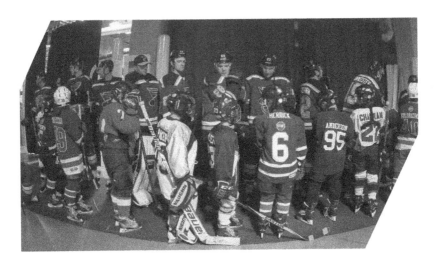

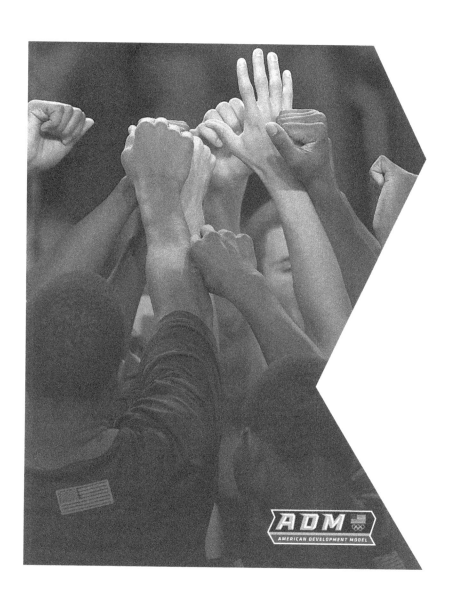

This publication is put forth by the United States Olympic Committee and the Department of Coaching Education in the Division of Sport Performance. For any inquiries on the American Development Model, please email CoachingEducation@usoc.org.

Further Reading

1) Roetert EP, Hainline B, Shell D. A complementary perspective of wellness related literacies. *Trans J Am Coll Sports Med* 2019;4:61–63.

2) Alosco ML, Kasimis AB, Stamm JM, et al. Age of first exposure to American football and long-term neuropsychiatric and cognitive outcomes. *Transl Psychiatry* 2017;7:e1236.

3) Belson K. Playing tackle football before 12 is tied to brain problems later. *New York Times*, September 19, 2017.

4) Policy Statement—American Academy of Pediatrics. Tackling in youth football: Council on Sports Medicine and Fitness. *Pediatrics* 2015;136:31419–e1430.

5) Chrisman SPD, Whitlock KB, Kroshus E, et al. Parents' perspectives regarding age restrictions for tackling in youth football. *Pediatrics* 2019;143:e20182402.

6) LaBella C. Youth tackle football: perception and reality. *Pediatrics* 2019;143:e21090519.

32 Legal and Insurance Concerns Following Concussion (I feel trapped in the Workers' Compensation system)

A 45-year-old male was walking over a wooden bridge for which coworkers had previously expressed safety concerns. One of the planks shifted and he fell, striking his right side on boulders. He did not strike his head, but his head jerked to the right and he immediately felt dizzy. He was diagnosed with rib fractures, a dislocated shoulder, and a concussion in the Emergency Department, and was discharged with instructions to follow up with a Workers' Compensation physician. One week later, he consulted with an orthopedic surgeon for management of his rib fractures and shoulder injury. Although he complained of headache, dizziness, poor memory, and neck pain, the orthopedic surgeon insisted he had no injuries to his head or neck, and he "should be fine."

He ultimately consulted with a neurologist who did not accept Workers' Compensation insurance because the wait time for neurologists within the system was six months, and he was noted to have abnormal eye movements.

What do you do now?

LEGAL AND INSURANCE CONCERNS FOLLOWING CONCUSSION

This case demonstrates several legal and insurance barriers to recovery from concussion. There are three elements of this case which must be considered carefully.

1) *Workers' Compensation*: Since this patient sustained an injury at work, to obtain medical treatment covered by insurance he is required to use Workers' Compensation insurance. Workers' Compensation providers must go through a credentialing process to participate, and all referrals for services must have a Workers' Compensation "C-4" referral form to justify the treatment. Even then, an independent Workers' Compensation board will determine whether medical services are necessary, and payment for such services is often lower than for commercial payers. Additionally, open legal actions involving patients injured at their workplace are common. Thus, most medical providers have little incentive to participate in the Workers' Compensation system unless it provides a source of substantial referrals. Furthermore, due to lower payments per patient, providers who do accept Workers' Compensation cases devote less time to each visit and may be more likely to order tests that generate additional income. Overall, these factors may limit patients' access to high-quality medical care.

"Independent medical examinations" (IMEs) are paid for by the Workers' Compensation board to prevent fraud in the system. Those who provide IMEs are typically providers paid by the board to interview and examine patients, review their records, and then determine if there is any ongoing medical problem. Payment for these examinations is also typically lower than payments by commercial payers for office visits. Furthermore, this process results in shorter visit times, and many patients say that the process can completely exclude an actual physical examination. Subtle neurological findings and nuanced details in the history may be missed, thus leading to a "negative" exam and a conclusion that no further medical treatment is necessary. Patients can appeal these decisions (which can be a lengthy process), so careful documentation by the provider is a critical part of the process.

Not only does Workers' Compensation require paperwork, even if patients cannot work, they may have to complete Family Medical Leave Act forms and disability insurance forms. Disability companies often require monthly updates, even when no significant change is expected within one month. Finally, human resources departments at individual companies may create their own forms. Workers' Compensation does not provide patients with a case manager or social worker, thus increasing the time patients must spend navigating the system. Patients with poor memory, dizziness, pain, or visual difficulties after a concussion are further compromised by this system.

In states with "no fault" auto insurance, individual providers do not need special credentials to work with injured patients. The patient and physician can both sign "provider assignment forms," and insurance companies will pay their standard fees for evaluation and treatment to any provider. These rates tend to be lower than commercial payers, but are consistently paid as long as the No Fault case is open, meaning that No Fault insurance agrees that ongoing medical treatment is warranted.

2) *Legal Concerns*: In this case, the injury happened on a bridge that the park was responsible for maintaining. Workers had already brought a concern about the bridge to management, which raises the question of whether the zoo has further financial liability for the patient's injury. Several studies have demonstrated that litigation is associated with more prolonged recovery of injury, including post-concussion. However, this association does not mean that patients are intentionally fabricating prolonged symptoms to get more money. The inherent stress caused by the legal process could also contribute to prolonged duration of symptoms.

The legal system generally requires objective data to support claims of financial liability. However, there are no objective biomarkers to measure the amount of neuronal injury from a concussion. This lack of objective data creates barriers to supporting claims of ongoing injury, which can hamper recovery. In such situations, a lawyer or plaintiff's expert physician may order a test that has not been validated (e.g., brain MRI with diffusion tensor imaging). A subsequent "positive" result both provides evidence of injury and potentially creates a "nocebo" effect, where the patient becomes convinced he or she is truly injured despite the lack of meaningful evidence.

The lack of objective biomarkers in concussion can also mean that patients are undercompensated for their injuries. Thus, it is even more important that practitioners clearly document abnormalities such as convergence insufficiency or abnormal smooth pursuit, and conduct a detailed cervical spine exam. Accurate documentation will also ensure that patients obtain appropriate coverage for necessary rehabilitation services and medications.

3) *Delays in treatment*: The patient had two musculoskeletal injuries in addition to his concussion injury, and Workers' Compensation and the legal system both prioritize treatment and payment for injuries that have objective testing correlates. Although early education regarding the trajectory of recovery after concussion may improve outcomes, such education is unlikely to occur in a 15-minute orthopedic surgery evaluation—especially when there are multiple injuries, many of which cannot be confirmed by objective testing.

Ultimately, workplace injuries and injuries that result in litigation must be managed and documented comprehensively, as with all injuries and clinical encounters. Appreciating the challenges of these circumstances may help prevent unnecessary suffering of patients and unnecessary testing by physicians.

TAKE-HOME POINTS

· Patients with workplace injuries must use Workers' Compensation insurance.
· Workers' Compensation insurance has an extremely limited network of providers, who are under increased time pressures when seeing such patients due to lower compensation rates.
· Participation in the legal process is associated with increased risk of prolonged symptoms; however, careful consideration of all factors that may impact recovery is crucial in each individual.
· When concussion presents with concurrent injuries, treatment of other injuries may be prioritized over concussion management, thereby delaying concussion recovery.
· To help ensure that patients obtain coverage for necessary rehabilitation and medical treatment, providers should carefully document any examination findings to explain ongoing symptoms (e.g., convergence insufficiency, standardized balance testing, thorough musculoskeletal examination).

Further Reading

1) Boden LI. Reexamining workers' compensation: a human rights perspective. *Am J Ind Med* 2012;55:483–486.

2) Matérne M, Strandberg T, Lundqvist LO. Risk markers for not returning to work among patients with acquired brain injury: a population-based register study. *J Occup Rehabil* 2019. doi: 10.1007/s10926-019-09833-6.

3) Hanks RA, Rapport LJ, Seagly K, et al. Outcomes after concussion recovery education: effects of litigation and disability status on maintenance of symptoms. *J Neurotrauma* 2019;36:554–558.

4) Tator CH, Davis HS, Dufort PA, et al. Postconcussion syndrome: demographics and predictors in 221 patients. *J Neurosurg* 2016;125:1206–1216.

PART IV

Long-Term Sequelae Considerations of Concussion

33 Mental Health Symptoms and Disorders Following Concussion (My husband says that I am always depressed)

A 40-year-old woman presented with complaints of depression. The patient was quite physically active in her youth, and played competitive rugby at the high school, college, and club levels for more than 10 years. She is uncertain how many concussions, if any, that she may have sustained, and she states that "having your bell rung" was always an accepted part of the game. She does state that she played a particularly aggressive form of rugby, and notes that she received frequent blows to the head from the knees and elbows of her opponents. For the past few years she has become increasingly depressed and socially withdrawn. Her husband believes that this has impacted the quality of their marriage and her relationship with their children.

What do you do now?

MENTAL HEALTH SYMPTOMS AND DISORDERS
FOLLOWING CONCUSSION

We understand that in the short term, behavioral sequelae are common following concussion. Indeed, most symptoms in the SCAT5 overlap with those attributable to anxiety and depression. Although acute mental health symptoms are common following concussion, these must be differentiated from a mental health disorder such as major depressive disorder or post-traumatic stress disorder. As discussed previously, most athletes recover from concussion within 7–10 days, but up to 20% may remain symptomatic longer. Some develop mental health disorders such as depression and anxiety, but others develop an array of symptoms in what is too often incorrectly diagnosed as post-concussion syndrome.

Proper management of sport-related concussion includes addressing any emerging mental health symptoms or disorders post-injury. Although there are as yet no prospective, longitudinal data to address long-term behavioral sequelae of concussion, emerging information suggests that depression risk is increased almost sixfold in former professional football players who have sustained more than five concussions. Other studies describe a threefold increase of depression following three or more sport-related concussions among retired football players. In former collegiate football players with a history of three or more concussions, there is a higher prevalence of moderate to severe depression in later life relative to the general population. However, the risk of suicide in former professional football players is significantly lower than in the general population.

There is also emerging information that long-term behavioral sequelae may be unrelated to concussion per se, but may reflect repetitive head impact exposure, especially among youth. Although these studies lack methodologic rigor, they suggest that first exposure to repetitive head impact before age 12 more strongly predicts long-term behavioral sequelae than first exposure after age 12. The hypothesis is that the brain is particularly vulnerable at a young age, and repetitive head impact exposure may affect brain myelination and underlying cytoarchitecture. How these changes affect development of mental health symptoms and disorders is not clear, nor is it clear if such sequelae are predictors of possible neurodegeneration.

At present, we cannot state that there is a causal relationship between either repetitive head impact exposure or concussion and the subsequent development of long-term mental health symptoms and disorders. These possible associations are important to explore. Nonetheless, providers should always perform a full differential diagnosis in patients who present with mental health symptoms and disorders, whether or not they sustained head injury in the past.

Athletes who have competed at a high level—including Olympic, professional, and collegiate athletes—may be specifically vulnerable to mental health symptoms and disorders independent of history of head injury. The subculture of sport differs from the general culture, and elite athletes have often subjected themselves to a life of overly intense discipline, sleep deprivation, overtraining, and repetitive injuries—sometimes serious. We also know that elite athletes have been victims of sexual and interpersonal violence; some evidence suggests that in some sports, the risk of such violence exceeds that of the general population.

Transition out of sport—especially forced transition, e.g., from injury or poor performance—is a strong risk factor for the development of mental health symptoms and disorders, especially among individuals who identify primarily as athletes. Former elite-level athletes are at risk for developing long-term symptoms of distress, sleep disturbance, anxiety, depression, and alcohol misuse.

Box 33.1 outlines risk factors for development of mental health symptoms and disorders in former athletes. The discerning clinician should perform a comprehensive evaluation of any former athlete who presents with mental health symptoms and disorders. Rather than assigning the risk to a category of former head trauma, a comprehensive protocol should always be followed.

Possible Risk Factors for the Development of Mental Health Symptoms and Disorder in Former Elite Athletes

- Family history of mental health symptoms and disorders
- Transition out of sport, especially forced retirement
- Chronic pain
- High level of athlete identity (and not personal identity otherwise)
- Lack of retirement planning
- Lower educational attainment because of sport
- Post-sport unemployment
- History of
  - Severe musculoskeletal injuries and/or multiple surgeries
  - Maladaptive perfectionism
  - Sexual/interpersonal violence
  - Alcohol or substance misuse/substance use disorder
  - Anabolic steroid use
  - Mental health symptoms and disorders
  - Multiple concussions
  - Repetitive head impact exposure

TAKE-HOME POINTS

- Mental health symptoms are common following acute concussion.
- Most individuals recover from acute mental health symptoms following concussion.
- A history or repetitive concussion and/or repetitive head impact exposure has been associated with the development of depression in later life.
- Former elite athletes are at risk of developing mental health symptoms and disorders independent of concussion and repetitive head impact exposure.
- When retired athletes present with mental health symptoms and disorders, the clinician should carefully assess risk factors.

Further Reading

1) Gouttebarge V, Castaldelli-Maia JM, Gorczynski P, et al. Occurrence of mental health symptoms and disorders in current and former elite athletes: a systematic review and meta-analysis. *Br J Sports Med* 2019;53:700–706.

2) Reardon CL, Hainline B, Aron CM, et al. Mental health in elite athletes: International Olympic Committee consensus statement. *Br J Sports Med* 2019;53:667–699.

3) Alosco ML, Stern RA. Youth exposure to repetitive head impacts from tackle football and long-term neurologic outcomes: a review of the literature, knowledge gaps and future directions, and societal and clinical implications. *Sem Ped Neurol* 2019;30:107–116.

4) Guskiewicz KM, Marshall SW, Bailes J, et al. Recurrent concussion and risk of depression in retired professional football players. *Med Sci Sports Exerc* 2007;39(6):903–909.

5) Kerr ZY, Thomas LC, Simon JE, et al. Association between history of multiple concussions and health outcomes among former college football players: 15-Year follow-up from the NCAA Concussion Study (1999–2001). *Am J Sports Med* 2018;46(7):1733–1741.

34 Cognitive Dysfunction Following Concussion (I keep forgetting things at work)

A 50-year-old man presented with complaints of short-term memory loss. He played multiple sports as a child, adolescent, and adult, including wrestling, martial arts, soccer, football, and tennis. He also was an extreme mountain biker, and states that he engaged in frequent high-risk biking and suffered several falls. He believes that he sustained many concussions, but always seemed to recover fully within two to three weeks. He played as an offensive lineman on the college football team. He has intermittent bouts of depression, but does not currently feel depressed. He admits to drinking three to five drinks per day, and has been smoking about one pack of cigarettes per day for the past 25 years. He has gained over 75 pounds since he graduated from college. He has hypertension and type 2 diabetes.

What do you do now?

COGNITIVE DYSFUNCTION FOLLOWING CONCUSSION

As with mental health symptoms and disorders, an emerging literature suggests a link between concussion, repetitive head impact exposure, and impaired cognition. It is important to differentiate impaired cognition from other mental health symptoms and disorders and other causes of dementia. There is no methodologically rigorous, prospective longitudinal study that can reveal causal connections between concussion, repetitive head impact exposure, and cognitive dysfunction of any etiology. That being said, it is important to understand emerging information.

In a study of 2,552 retired football players, those with three or more reported concussions had a fivefold increased prevalence of mild cognitive impairment and a threefold increased prevalence of reported significant memory problems, compared with retired football players without a history of concussion. Further, those who had Alzheimer's disease in this cohort had an earlier onset compared with the general population of American men.

There is also a suggested association between repetitive head impact exposure and later-life cognitive impairment. Because we have only recently developed direct ways of measuring head impact exposure using head accelerometers, prior exposure to repetitive head impacts must be estimated based on an index scale. This scale assesses retrospectively the threshold dose-response relationship between cumulative head impact index and risk for later life cognitive impairment, self-reported executive dysfunction, apathy, and depression. There is further emerging literature on possible correlations between multiple concussions, repetitive head impact exposure, or both and the development of Alzheimer's disease, chronic traumatic encephalopathy, and other neurodegenerative diseases. This subject will be discussed further in the final chapter.

As with mental health symptoms and disorders, any athlete who presents with cognitive impairment must undergo full evaluation for all causes of cognitive impairment, including underlying depression. Further, athletes with cognitive impairment and a history of concussion or repetitive head impact exposure should undergo evaluation of the

> **BOX 34.1. Differential Diagnosis Considerations in Former Contact/Collision Sport Athletes Who Present with Cognitive Decline**
>
> Undermanaged "post-concussion syndrome"
> Mental health symptoms and disorders
> Hypothalamic-pituitary dysfunction
> Metabolic syndrome and cerebral vasculopathy
> Cognitive impairment secondary to prior brain injury and limited
>   cognitive reserve
> Neurodegeneration

hypothalamic-pituitary axis, as pituitary dysfunction may adversely impact cognition and mood.

Some athletes may be at higher risk of vasculopathy and the metabolic syndrome. This subset could include athletes with a large body mass (such as former football linemen or wrestlers) or athletes who rapidly gain weight following retirement. These conditions are linked to vascular dementia.

Box 34.1 provides important differential diagnosis considerations when former athletes, especially those exposed to brain injury, present with cognitive impairment. The discerning clinician must evaluate for reversible causes of cognitive impairment, especially among those who present with "post-concussion syndrome" or mental health symptoms and disorders. In these individuals, cognitive impairment may result from unresolved persistent post-concussion symptoms or undermanaged mental health symptoms and disorders. A subset of patients may present with chronic cognitive impairment, but do not have progressive neurodegenerative disease. These individuals may have had prior brain injury and now are experiencing a lack of brain capacity to accommodate normal cognitive decline secondary to aging. Progressive dementia should never be simply assumed to be chronic traumatic encephalopathy, and even some dementing illnesses may stabilize or improve if they are secondary to underlying metabolic or pro-inflammatory conditions that affect vascular pathology.

· Cognitive decline has been associated with multiple concussions and repetitive head impact exposure.

· Cognitive decline may result from hypopituitarism, undermanaged post-concussion persistent symptoms, or mental health symptoms and disorders.

· Cognitive decline may be a relatively static phenomenon from prior brain injury.

· Cognitive decline may be the result of neurodegenerative disease.

· Cognitive decline should never be simply assumed to be the result of concussion or repetitive head impact exposure in former contact/collision sport athletes.

Further Reading

1) Montenigro PH, Alosco ML, Martin BM, et al. Cumulative head impact exposure predicts later-life depression, apathy, executive dysfunction, and cognitive impairment in former high school and college football players. *J Neurotrauma* 2017;34:328–340.

2) Guskiewicz KM, Marshall SW, Bailes J, et al. Association between recurrent concussion and late-life cognitive impairment in retired professional football players. *Neurosurg* 2005;57:719–726.

3) McInnes K, Friesen CL, MacKenzie DE, et al. Mild traumatic brain injury (mTBI) and chronic cognitive impairment: a scoping review. *PLoS One* 2017;12:e0174847.

35 Unmasking Neuropsychiatric Disorders Following Concussion

Part A: Unmasking Psychotic Disorders Following Concussion (Nick struck his head 8 months ago and now believes his brain has been hacked by the government.)

Nick, a 21-year-old college senior with migraines, sustained a possible concussion eight months ago after he collided with a door frame while walking to class with his eyes closed in an attempt to avoid bright lights. He had no acute symptoms, but over the next several months, he developed worsening headaches and increasing difficulty with concentration. He then began to hear distracting, random words and sounds. More recently, Nick has begun to hear an inner narrative with negative comments about his behavior, appearance, and academic performance, which he attributed to a government tracking device. Nick's parents report that he had no prior psychiatric issues, but struggled to fit in socially in college. He ultimately left school and returned home to complete his degree at a local community college. A psychiatrist diagnosed Nick with schizophrenia—a diagnosis his maternal grandfather was also given—but his parents believe he suffered a concussion that has caused his difficulties.

What do you do now?

UNMASKING PSYCHOTIC DISORDERS
FOLLOWING CONCUSSION

Psychosis can occur as a result of moderate to severe traumatic brain injury (TBI), but it is not an expected consequence of concussion. The DSM-5 defines psychotic disorders as characterized by symptoms in one or more of the following five domains: delusions, hallucinations, disorganized thinking, disorganized motor behavior, and negative symptoms (Table 35.1). The emergence of psychotic symptoms at any point after a concussion should always be taken seriously, as they may signal a more severe brain injury than was initially appreciated. Such patients may be experiencing an adverse effect of medications or other toxic-metabolic disturbance; they may be using substances to enhance athletic performance (stimulants, anabolic steroids) or for pleasure (cannabinoids); or they may be developing a major psychiatric disorder that will likely require long-term treatment (Table 35.2).

Post-traumatic psychosis refers to a specific syndrome of delusions and/or hallucinations with relative absence of negative symptoms that results from structural brain injury; it is not generally associated with concussion. Schizophrenia, in contrast, is diagnosed more often in patients with a history of concussion and more severe brain injuries. The reasons for this are

TABLE 35.1 **Key Features of Psychotic Disorders as Defined in DSM-5**

Delusions	· Fixed, false beliefs not amenable to change in light of conflicting evidence
Hallucinations	· Perception-like experiences that occur without external stimuli
Disorganized thinking	· Nonlinear speech/thought process, may jump between unrelated topics
Disorganized or abnormal motor behavior	· Impaired goal-directed motor behavior; includes catatonia
Negative symptoms	· Diminished emotional expression · Avolition · Asociality · Paucity of speech/thought

TABLE 35.2 **Differential Diagnosis of Psychotic Symptoms after Concussion**

Post-traumatic psychosis	· Prominent delusions and/or hallucinations · Relative absence of negative symptoms · Associated with moderate to severe brain injury · Can be associated with post-traumatic epilepsy
Toxic-metabolic disturbances	· Medication adverse effect (e.g., stimulants) · Delirium
Psychiatric illness	· Depression, mania, or PTSD with psychotic features · Substance misuse (e.g., cannabinoids, anabolic steroids) · Schizophrenia

unknown, but it is doubtful that concussion causes schizophrenia. Rather, the physiologic and psychological stress of a TBI may interact with underlying genetic vulnerabilities toward psychosis, thereby producing or unmasking a latent psychotic disorder. This stress-diathesis model is supported by data indicating that a family history of schizophrenia is a risk factor for developing schizophrenia after TBI.

Because family history of schizophrenia is also a risk factor for exposure to TBI—even in family members not diagnosed with schizophrenia—genetic and physiologic variations predisposing to schizophrenia also may increase the risk of concussion and other brain injuries. Early psychosis itself may place patients at greater risk of TBI via increased risk-taking and disorganized behavior, and rates of TBI of all severities and other accidental injuries are elevated in the year before a patient's first lifetime hospitalization for schizophrenia. However, recall bias in retrospective research studies is possible, as patients and families are more likely to identify and report histories of even very mild TBI in an attempt to make sense of a schizophrenia diagnosis.

In this case, the reported pre-head injury history of academic decline and the odd circumstances around the possible concussion itself (walking with eyes closed) suggest that Nick was beginning to experience prodromal symptoms of schizophrenia, and that his head injury occurred as a result of this process, rather than as a cause of it. The mild nature of the injury make it unlikely that he had post-traumatic psychosis due to structural brain injury. If he did experience mild post-concussive symptoms, they may have been an additional anxiety-provoking stressor that led to further psychiatric destabilization.

Schizophrenia is a devastating diagnosis; it is understandable that patients and families may seek out all alternative explanations (including identifying minor injuries and traumas as potential etiologic triggers) before accepting it. However, it is critical to address the underlying neurobiology of the disease and its associated psychosocial influencers, rather than focusing on a condition that is not causative or meaningfully contributory to patients' diagnoses and care plans.

TAKE-HOME POINTS

- Psychosis is not an expected consequence of concussion.
- Presence of psychotic symptoms after concussion should prompt immediate further evaluation for more severe brain injury, toxic-metabolic disturbances, and psychiatric illness.

Further Reading

1) Fujii D, Fujii DC. Psychotic disorder due to traumatic brain injury: analysis of case studies in the literature. *J Neuropsychiatry Clin Neurosci* 2012; 24:278–289.

2) Gurin L, Arciniegas DB. Psychotic disorders. In Silver JM, McAllister TW, Arciniegas DB (Eds.), 3rd edition, *Textbook of Traumatic Brain Injury*, Washington, DC: American Psychiatric Association, 2018, Chapter 22.

3) Molloy C, Conroy RM, Cotter DR, et al. Is traumatic brain injury a risk factor for schizophrenia? A meta-analysis of case-controlled population-based studies. *Schizophr Bull* 2011;37:1104–1110.

4) Currie A, Gorczynski P, Rice S, et al. Bipolar and psychotic disorders in elite athletes: a narrative review. *Br J Sports Med* 2019;53:746–753.

Part B: Unmasking Dementia Following Concussion (My wife thinks she is fine, but she can't remember anything.)

An 85-year-old woman presented with memory loss. Three weeks earlier she slipped and fell in her bathtub; she struck her occiput and lost consciousness. At the Emergency Department, her Glasgow Coma Scale was 15 and she complained of headache. She underwent a non-contrast head CT scan, which showed mild global atrophy and mild microvascular disease. Although her headache abated, she noticed persistent dizziness without vertigo. At follow-up evaluation three weeks later, her husband reported the new onset of short-term memory loss that seemed uncharacteristic for someone who was otherwise quite socially active and an avid reader of philosophy. The patient insisted she was fine. The neurological exam revealed a Mini-Mental State Exam of 25/30 and a subtle gait dyspraxia.

What do you do now?

UNMASKING DEMENTIA FOLLOWING CONCUSSION

The elderly are at increased risk of falls and subsequent head trauma due to the increased incidence of several conditions with age, including degenerative joint and spine disease, polyneuropathy, cervical myelopathy, and brain-mediated gait disorders. Although individuals aged 55 and older account for most hospitalizations from traumatic brain injury (TBI), the acute and sub-acute effects of concussion in this population are poorly understood. There is some evidence that prior TBIs, especially moderate/severe or multiple events, can predispose to later-life cognitive decline or neurodegenerative diseases such as Alzheimer's disease or chronic traumatic encephalopathy, but causal relationships remain speculative.

This patient functioned at a high level prior to her fall, and then seemingly declined more precipitously. In such situations, head trauma should not be presumed as the cause of the neurocognitive decline, and an appropriate diagnostic workup should be performed. In this case, the patient's further workup revealed mild hypertension, microvascular white matter changes noted on brain MRI, and an otherwise unremarkable metabolic profile. However, the brain volumetric and microvascular changes were prominent enough that one might have expected some prior neurocognitive decline. Her high level of functioning may have resulted from "cognitive reserve," a term used to describe individuals with neuropathologic brain changes but intact neurologic function. This concept of "resiliency" is thought to be mediated by high educational and occupational attainments and ongoing robust leisure activities later in life. This patient may have been functioning at the limit of her cognitive reserve before her fall. Thus, after the concussion, her brain could no longer compensate for the post-concussion vestibular dysfunction, leading to her seemingly precipitous decline.

Tables 35.3 and 35.4 show findings for various dementing illnesses that suggest diagnoses not caused by concussion. Formal neuropsychological evaluation can be extremely helpful in these situations, as the results may differentiate cognitive decline from mental health symptoms or disorders from maladaptive coping.

TABLE 35.3 Examination Findings Suggestive of Underlying Neurodegenerative Diseases

Examination Finding	Degenerative Syndrome
Amnestic deficits out of proportion to other abnormalities	Alzheimer's disease or mild cognitive impairment
Paratonia	Several dementias
Rigidity, masked facies, bradykinesia	Parkinson's disease, Lewy body dementia, multiple systems atrophy
Behavioral changes disproportional to memory loss, abnormal reflexes (e.g., snout, palmo-mental, glabellar tap, applause sign)	Frontotemporal dementia, chronic traumatic encephalopathy, or advanced dementias of any cause
Polyneuropathy	Amyloidosis
Atrophy and fasciculations in combination with hyper-reflexia	Amyotrophic lateral sclerosis and myeloradiculopathy
Chorea, tremor, other movement disorders	Disorders of the basal ganglia
Shuffling gait	Parkinsonian syndromes, normal pressure hydrocephalus

TABLE 35.4 Imaging Findings That Can Suggest a Diagnosis Other than Concussion

Imaging Finding	Degenerative Syndrome
Microhemorrhage, cortical superficial siderosis, microinfarcts, white matter hyperintensities, cortical thinning on MRI	Amyloid angiopathy
Microvascular disease and chronic strokes on CT or MRI	Vascular dementia
Communication hydrocephalus on CT or MRI	Normal pressure hydrocephalus

(*continued*)

TABLE 35.4 **Continued**

Imaging Finding	Degenerative Syndrome
Lobar atrophy and hypometabolism on FDG PET/MRI	Alzheimer's disease, frontotemporal dementia, and other specific degenerative syndromes
Mesial temporal sclerosis on MRI	Epilepsy
Cerebellar atrophy	Chronic alcoholism, cerebellar degenerative diseases
Inferior frontal, anterior temporal, occipital gliosis	Previous history of more severe brain trauma
Basal ganglia signal change	Wilson's disease, Huntington's disease

TAKE-HOME POINTS

- Concussion may unmask or worsen underlying dementia, but does not cause acute dementia.
- Multiple concussions or moderate/severe traumatic brain injury may lead to dementia many years later.
- Thorough neuropsychological evaluation can help differentiate among underlying dementing illnesses, mental health symptoms/disorders, and maladaptive responses.
- Patients who develop dementia following concussion should undergo a thorough neurologic exam and diagnostic workup to assess for any underlying neurodegenerative or toxic/metabolic diseases.

Further Reading

1) Levin HS, Mattis S, Ruff RM, et al. (1987). Neurobehavioral outcome following minor head injury: a three-center study. *J Neurosurg* 1987;66:234–243.
2) Goldstein FC, Levin HS, Goldman WP, et al. Cognitive and neurobehavioral functioning after mild versus moderate traumatic brain injury in older adults. *J Int Neuropsychol Soc* 2001;7:373–383.
3) Papa L, Mendes ME, Braga CF. Mild traumatic brain injury among the geriatric population. *Curr Transl Geriatr Exp Gerontol Rep* 2012;1:135–142.
4) Stern Y. Cognitive reserve in ageing and Alzheimer's disease. *Lancet Neurol* 2013;11:1006–1012.

36 Chronic Traumatic Encephalopathy (My husband's behavior is increasingly erratic)

A 55-year-old man presented with complaints of increasingly erratic behavior and memory loss. He was accompanied by his wife, and had poor insight as to why he was being evaluated. His past medical history is notable for binge alcohol drinking and anabolic steroid use. He played multiple sports as a child, including tackle football and soccer. He became increasingly specialized in tackle football in high school and had a rather successful career as a collegiate and professional football player. Upon retirement, he started his own company selling auto parts. Although his business was originally successful, he became increasingly suspicious of his business partners. He sometimes arrived at work after binge drinking, and the business eventually imploded. He became increasingly forgetful in all spheres of life, and frequently became lost while driving a car. More recently he developed violent outbursts, and his wife has become concerned about her safety.

What do you do now?

CHRONIC TRAUMATIC ENCEPHALOPATHY

Chronic traumatic encephalopathy (CTE) has become a household term and is now the center of a polarizing debate. There are those who believe that the causes of CTE have been firmly established, and that tackle football definitely causes CTE. At the other end of the spectrum, there are those who believe that CTE is not a distinct neurologic condition but has mixed features of other neurologic diseases. The quest for truth lies somewhere in between.

Historical Perspectives

The term "chronic traumatic encephalopathy" was first used in 1942 to describe a single case report. Critchley also used the term CTE in 1949, but he later modified this to "chronic progressive traumatic encephalopathy." There were previous case reports of boxers who had a neurologic condition called "dementia pugilistica" or "punch drunk syndrome." Critchley and others did not make a clear correlation between dementia pugilistica, punch drunk syndrome, and CTE. Indeed, the scientific literature was essentially silent on all of these conditions until the twenty-first century. Standard textbooks of neurology and sports medicine did not discuss CTE until after the first decade of the twenty-first century.

A single case report, published in 2005, described a "new" neurological condition called CTE. This report provided a clinical description of progressive behavioral and cognitive dysfunction, with neuropathology of hyperphosphorylated tau, in a pattern that seemed distinct from other tauopathies such as Alzheimer's disease. More case reports, case series, and articles on convenience samples followed, all describing a clinical pattern of some combination of behavioral, motor, and cognitive decline with distinct neuropathologic findings.

An accepted neuropathologic criterion for the diagnosis of CTE emerged in February 2015. The inaugural consensus meeting regarding CTE neuropathology was held jointly by the National Institute of Neurological Disorders and Stroke (NINDS) and the National Institute of Biomedical Imaging and Bioengineering (NIBIB). This consensus meeting described the pathognomonic lesion of CTE as "an accumulation of abnormal hyperphosphorylated tau (p-tau) in neurons and astroglia distributed around small blood vessels at the depths of cortical sulci and in an irregular pattern." Although this is the only pathognomonic lesion accepted as the criterion for CTE, there remain less formal criteria in the scientific literature and the lay press, including descriptions of CTE in stages.

Unfortunately, the intent of the joint NINDS/NIBIB is too often overlooked by clinicians, researchers, the media, and attorneys. Too many have assumed that the diagnostic criteria of CTE is now a settled manner. However, the consensus paper authors (Reference 3) made the following important points:

- Further consensus meetings will address validation of the criteria among a wider group of neuropathologists using cases submitted from multiple sources.
- Further meetings will address the identification of comorbid CTE when other neurodegenerative diseases and other diseases are present.
- Additional research will be necessary to determine the contribution of p-tau and other pathologies to the development of clinical symptoms of CTE.
- The incidence and prevalence of CTE remain unknown.
- This first consensus conference represents the first step along the path to standardizing the neuropathology of CTE and paving the way for future determinations of specific clinical symptomatology and refinements in clinical diagnosis.

The scientific literature and media coverage of CTE has been primarily driven by a convenience sample of donated brains to a single institution. A clear majority of these brains, primarily from former professional football players, have confirmed CTE. However, the incidence and prevalence of CTE remain unknown, in both the general population and former athletes. There is emerging information that CTE can develop in individuals with no known history of concussion or repetitive brain injury, leading some to suggest that CTE may be associated with risk factors other than brain injury.

Clinical Manifestations

There are no universally accepted clinical criteria for diagnosing CTE, and the diagnosis can only be made post mortem. Subtypes of CTE have been described, with any combination of the following: (1) behavioral problems, including impulsivity, depression, anxiety, violence, apathy, and paranoia; (2) global cognitive decline; and (3) loss of motor control, with features of parkinsonism. The search for objective biomarkers is ongoing, with preliminary evidence that differences in tau distribution between CTE and other tauopathies may be discerned using positron emission tomography scans.

Any individual (athlete or non-athlete) who presents with progressive changes in any combination of behavior, cognition, and motor dysfunction should undergo a complete neurologic evaluation. This evaluation should be searching for treatable neurologic conditions, including "post-concussion syndrome" and mental health disorders. If the diagnosis is presumed CTE or a neurodegenerative condition such as Alzheimer's disease or another tauopathy, management should also focus on symptom control.

Gap Analysis

Scientific understanding of CTE is still in its infancy, and we have the following knowledge gaps:

- We do not understand the specific risk factors for CTE.
- We do not know if there is a genetic predisposition to CTE.
- We do not know the incidence and prevalence of CTE in athletes who have participated in contact/collision sports.
- We do not know the incidence and prevalence of CTE in the general population.
- We do not understand the relationship of CTE to other neurodegenerative conditions and other neurological diseases.
- We do not know if all cases of CTE are progressive.
- We do not know if there is a relationship between the clinical features of CTE and tau pathology.

The knowledge gaps described for CTE are similar to the knowledge gaps of all tauopathies. As emerging information about this condition is produced, we should develop policies in sport that emphasize the personal and societal benefits of sport as well as player safety in sport.

· Although CTE was first described in 1949, it did not become a noticeable sports medicine or neurologic issue of concern until the twenty-first century.

· CTE is a tauopathy with distinct neuropathologic distribution of hyperphosphorylated tau.

· CTE has been described clinically as any combination of dysfunction in behavioral, cognitive, and motor domains.

· CTE has been associated with athletes who have a history of prior brain injury, including concussion and repetitive head impact exposure.

· CTE can only be diagnosed post-mortem.

· There are considerable gaps in our knowledge regarding the incidence, prevalence, and cause of CTE.

Further Reading

1) Hainline B, Stern RA. Future directions. In Hainline B, Stern RA (Eds.), *Sports Neurology*, San Diego: Elsevier BV, 2018, pp 473–480.

2) D'Ascanio S, Alosco ML, Stern RA. Chronic traumatic encephalopathy: clinical presentation and in vivo diagnosis. In Hainline B, Stern RA (Eds.), *Sports Neurology*, San Diego: Elsevier BV, 2018, pp 281–296.

3) McKee AC, Cairns NJ, Dickson DW, et al. The first NINDS/NIBIB consensus meeting to define neuropathological criteria for the diagnosis of chronic traumatic encephalopathy. *Acta Neuropathol* 2016;131:75–86.

4) Ling H, Holton JL, Shaw K, et al. Histological evidence of chronic traumatic encephalopathy in a large series of neurodegenerative diseases. *Acta Neuropathol* 2015;130:891–893.

5) Iverson GL, Gardner AJ, McCrory P, et al. A critical review of chronic traumatic encephalopathy. *Neurosci Biobehav Rev* 2015;56:276–293.

Index

Note: Tables and boxes are indicated by *t* and *b* following the page number
For the benefit of digital users, indexed terms that span two pages (e.g., 52–53) may, on occasion, appear on only one of those pages.

CBTI (cognitive behavioral therapy for insomnia), 94–95
Center for Neurologic Study-Lability Scale (CNS-LS), 114
Centers for Disease Control and Prevention, 4–5
cervicalgia. *See* neck pain
cervical spine injury, 34–35
  assessment for, 34
  emergency action plan for spinal stabilization, 34–35, 35*b*
  examination for, 153*b*
  neck pain, 152
  "red flags" for cervical spine injury, 34*b*, 34
Child Sport Concussion Assessment Tool-5 (Child SCAT5), 21
chronic traumatic encephalopathy (CTE), 50, 178–79, 241
  clinical manifestations of, 243
  cognitive dysfunction, 226, 227
  dementia, 236, 237*t*
  historical perspectives of, 241–42
  knowledge gaps, 243
  subtypes of, 243
circadian dysregulation, 94–95, 95*t*
CNS-LS (Center for Neurologic Study-Lability Scale), 114
coaches and athletic trainers, 10–11, 170–71
  educating, 39*b*, 48, 171, 178
  influence of, 162
  relationship with health professionals, 162–63
cocoon therapy, 70
cognitive behavioral therapy for insomnia (CBTI), 94–95
cognitive dysfunction, 147, 225
  clinical profiles that can impair cognitive function, 148*b*
  cognitive tests, 148
  differential diagnosis, 226, 227*b*, 227
  evaluating, 226–27
  increased risk, 226

  neuropsychology referrals, 149
  repetitive head impact exposure and, 226
  subset of athletes at higher risk, 227
  susceptible domains, 148
computed tomography (CT)
  "red flags" for ordering a brain CT scan, 5–6, 6*b*
  suggesting diagnosis other than concussion, 75, 237*t*
concussion
  anxiety following, 105
  attention-deficit/hyperactivity disorder and, 117
  autonomic dysfunction following, 128
  catastrophic brain injury *vs.*, 38
  cervical spine injury and, 34
  chronic traumatic encephalopathy, 241
  coaches and athletic trainers, 162–163
  cognitive dysfunction and, 148, 226–27
  definitions, 4–5, 5*b*, 46
  dementia following, 235–38
  depression following, 102–103
  in Emergency Department, 4–5
  emotional dysregulation following, 112–13
  evolution of symptoms, 46
  expectation management, 83
  on field of play, 10
  hiding, 157
  legal and insurance concerns following, 211
  mental health symptoms and disorders, 219
  migraine and other headache disorders following, 97
  mild traumatic brain injury *vs.*, 4, 83
  multiple, and subsequent retirement from sport, 165
  neck pain following, 151
  objective biomarkers, 73
  oculomotor dysfunction and, 133
  pituitary dysfunction and, 137
  prolonged recovery, 50
  protective equipment and, 174

psychotic disorders following, 229
return to learning, 53
return to play, 69
second impact syndrome *vs.*, 41
shift in diagnosis and management of,
ix, 70–71
sleep disorder and, 93
vestibular dysfunction and, 124
women and, 141
youth tackle football and, 177
Concussion Assessment, Research and
Educational Consortium (CARE), 76
Concussion in Sport Group, 4–5, 5*b*, 70,
152, 166, 171
Concussion Recognition Tool 5, 10–11,
11*b*, 30
Council on Sports Medicine and
Fitness, 178–79
Critchley, M., 241
CT. *See* computed tomography
CTE. *See* chronic traumatic encephalopathy

dementia, 235–38
cognitive dysfunction, 226, 227
concept of "resiliency," 236
findings suggestive of underlying
neurodegenerative diseases, 237*t*
imaging findings suggesting diagnosis
other than concussion, 237*t*
risks for elderly, 236
depression, 101–102
affective lability, 114
chronic traumatic encephalopathy, 243
cognitive dysfunction, 226–27
criteria for major depressive
disorder, 102*t*
depressive symptoms *vs.* major depressive
disorder *vs.* brain injury, 102–3
management of, 103, 103*t*
mental health symptoms and
disorders, 220
migraine and other headache disorders,
98–99, 99*b*

pituitary dysfunction, 138
transition out of sport, 102
diagnosis threat, 83, 85*t*
*Diagnostic and Statistical Manual of Mental
Disorders*, 5th edition (DSM-5), 90,
102*t*, 231
diffusion tensor imaging (DTI), 75
disability insurance, 213–14

electroencephalography (EEG), 76*t*, 119–20
emotional dysregulation,
affective lability, 112, 112–13*t*, 114
irritability, 112, 112–13*t*, 114
pathologic laughing and crying, 112–13,
112–13*t*
epilepsy, 232*t*, 237*t*
expectation management, 48
best practices for preventing persistent
post-concussive symptoms, 85*t*
diagnostic terminology and diagnosis
threat, 83, 85*t*
early education and empowerment,
84–85, 85*t*
risk factors for prolonged post-concussive
symptoms, 83–84, 84*t*
symptom assessment and management,
85, 85*t*

Family Medical Leave Act, 213–14
Fifth International Conference on
Concussion in Sport, 46, 47*b*, 90
fludrocortisone, 131*t*
fluid biomarkers, 77, 77*t*
fMRI (functional brain MRI), 76, 170
follicle-stimulating hormone, 138*b*
Football Development Model Council, 180
frontotemporal dementia, 237*t*
functional brain MRI (fMRI), 76, 170

genetic biomarkers, 77–78, 78*t*
Glasgow Coma Scale, 4, 4*t*
glial fibrillary acidic protein (GFAP), 75, 77
growth hormone, 138*b*

otolith dysfunction, 123
semicircular canal dysfunction, 123
vestibular migraine, 123–24
white matter abnormalities, 123–24
vestibular migraine, 123–24
Vestibular/Ocular Motor Screening
    (VOMS), 124–25, 124*t*
video-oculography, 134

white matter abnormalities, 75,
    123–24, 123*t*
Wilson's disease, 237*t*
women and concussion, 141
    gender-based/sociocultural differences,
        143, 144, 145*t*
    injury mechanisms, 143–44
    pituitary dysfunction, 137
    post-concussive symptoms, 144, 145*t*
    prevalence of, 143, 145*t*

recovery, 144–45, 145*t*
sex-based differences, 143–44, 145*t*
Workers' Compensation insurance,
    213–14, 215
    factors limiting access to high-quality
        medical care, 213
    independent medical examinations, 213
    No Fault insurance, 214
    paperwork, 213–14

youth tackle football, 177
    American Development Model, 179–80,
        181–208
    current lack of physical literacy, 178
    Football Development Model
        Council, 180
    importance of physical literacy, 178
    movement to ban, 179
    study of risks associated with, 178–79